Workbook and Lab Manual for Sonography:

Introduction to Normal Structure and Function

Workbook and Lab Manual for Sonography:
Introduction to Normal Structure and Function

Fifth edition

Reva Arnez Curry, PhD, RTR, RDMS, FSDMS
Vice-President of Instruction and Learning Services
Academic Services
Delta College
University Center, Michigan

Marilyn Prince, BS, MPH, RDMS, RVT
Ultrasound Consultant
Retired Ultrasound Supervisor
Department of Radiology
Emory University Hospital

Atlanta, Georgia

ELSEVIER

Elsevier
3251 Riverport Lane
St. Louis, Missouri 63043

Notice

Practitioners and researchers must always rely on their own experience and knowledge in evaluating and using any information, methods, compounds or experiments described herein. Because of rapid advances in the medical sciences, in particular, independent verification of diagnoses and drug dosages should be made. To the fullest extent of the law, no responsibility is assumed by Elsevier, authors, editors or contributors for any injury and/or damage to persons or property as a matter of products liability, negligence or otherwise, or from any use or operation of any methods, products, instructions, or ideas contained in the material herein.

Previous editions copyrighted 2017, 2016, 2011, 2009, 2007.

Executive Content Strategist: Sonya Seigafuse
Senior Content Development Manager: Luke Held
Content Development Specialist: John Tomedi, Spring Hollow Press
Publishing Services Manager: Deepthi Unni
Project Manager: Srividhya Vidhyashankar

Printed in United States of America

Last digit is the print number: 9   8   7   6   5   4

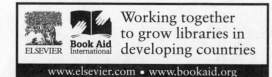

Contributors

Myka Bussey-Campbell, M.Ed.
Program Coordinator
Diagnostic Medical Sonography
Diagnostic and Therapeutic Sciences
Georgia Southern University - Armstrong Campus
Savannah, Georgia

Aaron Matthew Chandler, BA, RDMS, RVT
Lead Sonographer
Ultrasound, Imaging Department
Alta Bates Summit Medical Center
Oakland, California
Clinical Instructor
Diagnostic Medical Sonography Program
Gurnick Academy of Medical Arts
San Mateo, California

Reva Arnez Curry, Ph.D.
Vice-President of Instruction and Learning Services
Academic Services
Delta College
University Center, Michigan

Tiana V. Curry-McCoy, PhD, MPH, MPA
MS-CLS Research Program Director
Department of Undergraduate Health Professions-
    Clinical Laboratory Science
College of Allied Health Sciences
Augusta University
Associate Member of Vascular Biology Center
Augusta, Georgia

Kacey Davis, M.Ed., BSRS, AS
Program Director
Diagnostic Medical Sonography
Assistant Professor
Diagnostic Medical Sonography
Albany State University
Albany, Georgia

Amy T. Dela Cruz, MS, BMME
Program Director
Medical Sonography
South Piedmont Community College
Monroe, North Carolina

Yonella Demars, BS, MSRS
Director, Diagnostic Medical Sonography
Radiation Sciences
Virginia Commonwealth University
Richmond, Virginia

Yvonne Z. Dillon, BSRS, M.Ed., RDMS
Sonography Clinical Coordinator/ Lecturer
Department of Diagnostic and Therapeutic Sciences
Georgia Southern University
Savannah, Georgia

Tara Renee Edwards, B.S, CVT Certificate
Cardiac Sonographer IV
Echocardiography Lab
Emory University Hospital
Atlanta, Georgia

Cheryl B. Grant, MS
Chief Sonographer
Ultrasound
WellStar AMC-Downtown
Atlanta, Georgia

Joy Guthrie, PhD., RDMS, RDCS, RVT
Advanced Practice Sonographer/ Program Director
Ultrasound/Cardiology
Community Regional Medical Center
Fresno, California

Nancy Leahy, AAS, BA, MA
Austin, Texas

Wayne Charles Leonhardt, BA, RDMS, RVT
Master Scanning Laboratory Vascular Instructor
Diagnostic Medical Sonography Program
Gurnick Academy of Medical Arts
San Mateo, California
Sonographer
Ultrasound
Mission Imaging Services
Asheville, North Carolina

Peggy Ann Malzi Bizjak, MBA, RDMS, CRA, RT(R) (M)
Radiology Manager, Ultrasound Division (Retired)
University of Virginia Health System
Charlottesville, Virginia
Adjunct Faculty, Diagnostic Medical Sonography
  Program
Health and Sciences Division
Piedmont Virginia Community College
Charlottesville, Virginia

Lily Ann Oberhelman, BSRS, M.Ed, RDMS, RVT
Staff Sonographer
General Ultrasound Department
St. Joseph's/Candler Hospital System
Savannah, Georgia
Part-time Faculty
Department of Diagnostic and Therapeutic Sciences
Georgia Southern University
Savannah, Georgia

Marilyn Prince, BS, MPH, RDMS, RVT
Ultrasound Consultant
Emory University
Atlanta, Georgia

Mitzi Roberts, Ed.D., RT(R), RDMS, RDCS
Faculty
Division of Allied Health
Baptist Memorial College of Health Sciences
Memphis, Tennessee

Lisa Strohl, BS, RT(R), RDMS, RVT
Remote Clinical Education Specialist—Ultrasound
Clinical Education and IT Solutions
GE Healthcare
Wauwatosa, Wisconsin

Avian L. Tisdale, B.S., M.D., MBA
Physician
Pediatrics
Night Light Urgent Care Pediatrics
Sugar Land, Texas

Rita Udeshi, B.S., ARDMS (OB/GYN/RVT/AB/AE/PS)
Children's Healthcare of Atlanta
Radiology Hospital
Atlanta, Georgia

Cheryl Vance, MA, RT, RDMS
CEO
C&D Advance Consultants, LLC
San Antonio, Texas

Kimberly B. Williams, RDMS, AB, OB, B
Sonographer
Ultrasound
Emory University Hospital Midtown, Atlanta
Georgia

Contents

SECTION I: CLINICAL APPLICATIONS

Chapter 1 Before, During, and After the Ultrasound Examination, **1**
Chapter 2 Ultrasound Instrumentation: "Knobology," Imaging Processing, and Storage, **16**
Chapter 3 General Patient Care, **20**
Chapter 4 Introduction to Ergonomics and Sonographer Safety, **22**

SECTION II: SONOGRAPHIC APPROACH TO UNDERSTANDING ANATOMY

Chapter 5 Interdependent Body Systems, **24**
Chapter 6 Anatomy Layering and Sectional Anatomy, **26**
Chapter 7 Embryology, **48**
Chapter 8 Introduction to Laboratory Values, **59**

SECTION III: ABDOMINAL SONOGRAPHY

Chapter 9 The Abdominal Aorta, **61**
Chapter 10 The Inferior Vena Cava, **70**
Chapter 11 The Portal Venous System, **81**
Chapter 12 The Liver, **91**
Chapter 13 The Biliary System, **104**
Chapter 14 The Pancreas, **116**
Chapter 15 The Urinary and Adrenal Systems, **131**
Chapter 16 Abdominal Vasculature, **151**
Chapter 17 The Spleen, **159**
Chapter 18 The Gastrointestinal System, **168**

SECTION IV: PELVIC SONOGRAPHY

Chapter 19 The Male Pelvis: Prostate Gland and Seminal Vesicles Sonography, **179**
Chapter 20 The Female Pelvis, **186**

SECTION V: OBSTETRIC AND NEONATAL SONOGRAPHY

Chapter 21 First Trimester Obstetrics (0 to 12 Weeks), **206**
Chapter 22 Second and Third Trimester Obstetrics (13 to 42 Weeks), **217**
Chapter 23 High-Risk Obstetrics, **236**
Chapter 24 Fetal Echocardiography, **241**
Chapter 25 The Neonatal Brain, **251**
Chapter 26 The Thyroid and Parathyroid Glands, **260**
Chapter 27 Breast Sonography, **270**
Chapter 28 Scrotal and Penile Sonography, **282**

SECTION VI: SPECIALTY SONOGRAPHY

Chapter 29 Pediatric Echocardiography, **293**
Chapter 30 Adult Echocardiography, **309**
Chapter 31 Vascular Technology, **324**

SECTION VII: ADVANCES IN SONOGRAPHY

Chapter 32 3D/4D/5D Sonography, **333**
Chapter 33 Interventional and Intraoperative Ultrasound, **342**
Chapter 34 Musculoskeletal Sonography, **349**
Chapter 35 Pediatric Sonography, **360**

Instructions for Students

Dear Students,

The purpose of this laboratory manual is to guide you in studying concepts presented in the textbook *Sonography: Introduction to Normal Structure and Function.*

This laboratory manual:

■ was written to be completed either independently during private study or with a student partner in a laboratory setting.

■ is built around the six levels of cognitive learning described in Bloom's taxonomy: memorization, comprehension, application, analysis, evaluation, and synthesis.

■ has been developed to help you learn sonographic anatomy, basic physiology, and image analysis through a progression from simple to complex, that is, from memorization of key words to comprehension of learning objectives, application of key concepts, analysis of images and illustrations, synthesis of chapter subheadings, and evaluation of the chapters.

Each chapter of the laboratory manual is structured to follow Bloom's taxonomy of six cognitive domains, with subsections that correlate with each cognitive level. This means that each section of the chapter "builds" on the previous one, just as each of Bloom's domains build on the previous one. The domains address memorization (knowledge), comprehension, application, analysis, evaluation, and synthesis, as shown in the chart below.

Bloom's Taxonomy Domain	Definition	Example
Memorization	Memorize facts, figures	Memorize key words, measure organs and vessels
Comprehension	Restate facts or concepts in your own words	Answer objectives in your own words
Application	Applying what you've learned in a new way	Draw, sketch, or label an organ and its parts

Bloom's Taxonomy Domain	Definition	Example
Analysis	Compare and contrast, note differences	Differentiate the normal appearance of organs and structures on sonographic images
Evaluation	Assess what has been learned, determine its value	Appraise the information presented and judge its value
Synthesis	Create something "new" from what has been learned	Write a technical impression

Bloom's Taxonomy is featured on several short You Tube videos that explain the concept. "Bloom's Taxonomy: Structuring the Learning Journey" is briefly described on You Tube: Sprouts at the following link: https://www.youtube.com/watch?time_continue=2&v=ayefSTAnCR8&feature=emb_title.

USING THE LABORATORY MANUAL

Before you begin each chapter, make sure you have read and studied the corresponding chapter in the *Sonography* textbook. To complete the laboratory manual chapters, you will need the following items:

■ The *Sonography* textbook and notes from the reading

■ Pen, colored pencils, or highlighters, and a notebook

■ Anatomy and physiology notes from other previous courses may be helpful as well.

The following suggestions will help you use optimize the use of this manual:

1. Quickly skim through the chapter in the laboratory manual. Open your textbook to the corresponding chapter. Note the exercises in the laboratory manual are designed to stimulate your learning of the concepts presented in the textbook.

2. Bloom's taxonomy domains are presented in sequential order in each chapter. Only appropriate domains are included.

3. Do the exercises in sequential order.

4. Write the answers in your notebook.

5. Write in the margin questions that you may have as you work through the exercises. Make a list of your questions, answer them as best you can, then check your answers with your instructor. What additional information did your instructor provide? How was it helpful to you? (This type of reflection will help you prepare for quizzes and tests.)

6. This manual contains unlabeled images and illustrations from every chapter in the textbook to test your comfort level with sonograms and identifying anatomy. Make sure you understand the images that are presented. Can you identify structures without labels? Do you know how to describe them? If you're still confused about the images presented in the manual, go back and reread the section in the textbook. We encourage you to color the structures on the illustrations to better differentiate the anatomy.

7. Make sure you understand which things in the text are important to your instructor. Think of these as guidelines. Write down these guidelines and refer to them as you study. This technique should help you prepare for major tests on the material.

8. Allow enough time for review and reflection at the end of the laboratory chapter. What did you learn that you did not know before? How can this help you improve your learning of normal structural anatomy and physiology?

Sonography is an exciting and challenging profession. We wish you the best in your education and career.

Reva Arnez Curry and Marilyn Prince

1 Before, During, and After the Ultrasound Exam

I. MEMORIZATION EXERCISE

1. Write the key words in your notebook or on note cards. Write the words on one side of the notepaper and then write the definitions on the opposite side of the page or on the back of the paper. If using note cards, write the key word on the front and the definition on the back. *This step should be completed before the lab session begins.*

   Memorize the key word definitions silently for 5 minutes, then work with a lab partner and identify the words for which you still need help. List the words here. Add additional rows if needed.

2. Review the patient positions in your textbook and write them in your notebook. Take turns correctly identifying the patient positions as demonstrated by you and your lab partner. (You may need a floor mat and to wear casual clothes to do this exercise.)

II. COMPREHENSION EXERCISE

1. Work with a lab partner to complete this exercise. You will need to write here or in your notebook. First, change each objective into a question.

   Example: "Explain the roles of the sonographer and sonologist in the ultrasound procedure" becomes "What are the roles of the sonographer and sonologist in the ultrasound procedure?"

Next, write a short answer to the question just created.

   Example: "A sonographer takes the patient history, explains the sonographic exam, performs the sonographic exam, and writes a technical observation of the images produced. A sonologist is a physician who assesses the images and dictates an interpretive report, which can include a definitive diagnosis or differential diagnoses."

   Highlight or circle any part of your answers about which you are unsure, and check the answers in your textbook. If you are still unsure of the answers, put a question mark next to the answer(s) for the review session of the lab.

III. APPLICATION EXERCISE

1. In your notebook, list the sources of hepatitis B virus/HIV transmission and how the transmission can occur. Write ways in which your exposure to hepatitis B virus/HIV can be reduced. Be as specific as possible. Ask your lab partner to critique your work. What did you miss?

2. Routine Inpatient Chart Review. Briefly review the inpatient charts in Box 1-1 and circle the diagnostic examinations. Compare and contrast inpatient chart items with items in the obstetrics, baby, rehabilitation, and psychiatry charts. What are the major similarities and differences?

BOX 1-1

Routine Inpatient Chart

1. Preadmission and admission forms
2. Consent forms for examinations and treatments
3. Living will
4. Physician's orders
5. Discharge assessment, planning and summary sheets
6. Emergency room records
7. Patient care plans and problem lists
8. Laboratory and Radiology report sections
9. Nursing transfer summary
10. History and physical examination reports
11. Progress notes
12. Consultation reports
13. Patient teaching record
14. Discharge instructions to patient
15. Specialty procedure reports
16. Operative reports and records (Pre-, peri- and post op)
17. Labor and Delivery reports
18. Pathology
19. Post-anesthesia record
20. Endoscopy report
21. Medical Intensive Care Unit reports
22. ECG/EKG rhythm strips
23. EEG
24. Antibody ID and allergy report
25. Nutrition reports
26. Fall risk
27. Cardiopulmonary resuscitation record
28. Transfer order sheet and reports from outside medical facilities and/or EMS
29. Medication administration record
30. Nursing care record
31. Critical care flow sheet
32. Neurologic assessment sheet
33. Neurologic checklist
34. Intake-output chart
35. Observation checklist for patients in seclusion or on suicide precautions form
36. Restraint record

Chapter **1**   **Before, During, and After the Ultrasound Exam**

IV. IMAGE ANALYSIS EXERCISE

1. Label the regional divisions of the abdomen.

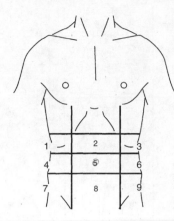

1 _____

2 _____

3 _____

4 _____

5 _____

6 _____

7 _____

8 _____

9 _____

Figure 1-3 in the textbook

2. Label the abdominal quadrants.

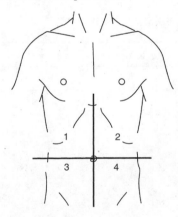

1 _____

2 _____

3 _____

4 _____

Figure 1-3 in the textbook

3. Label the anatomical planes and directions.

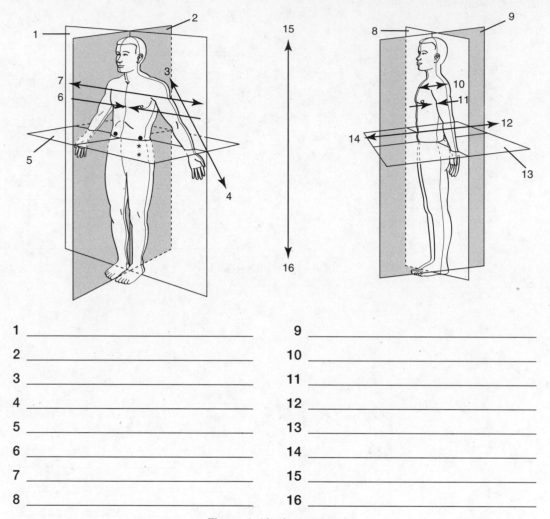

1	_____	9	_____
2	_____	10	_____
3	_____	11	_____
4	_____	12	_____
5	_____	13	_____
6	_____	14	_____
7	_____	15	_____
8	_____	16	_____

Figure 1-4 in the textbook

4. For each view shown in Figures 1-5, 1-6, and 1-7 from the textbook, identify on the pie shape the appropriate directional terms (e.g., posterior/anterior, superior/inferior, lateral/medial, right/left, right or left lateral) as indicated by numbers 1, 2, 3, and 4 on each wedge.

Sagittal Scanning Plane
2 sound wave approaches are possible
Anterior or Posterior

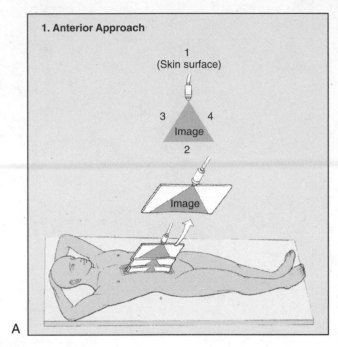
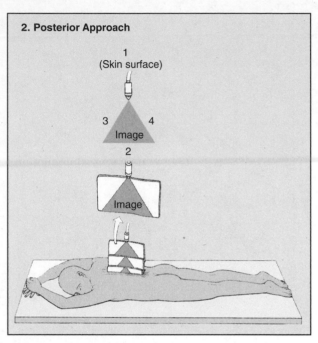

1 _____
2 _____
3 _____
4 _____

1 _____
2 _____
3 _____
4 _____

Figure 1-5 in the textbook

Coronal Scanning Plane
2 sound wave approaches are possible
Left lateral or Right lateral

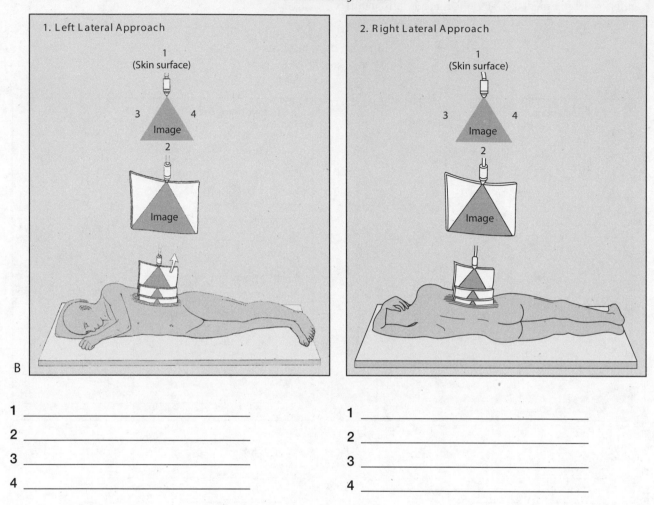

1 _____
2 _____
3 _____
4 _____

1 _____
2 _____
3 _____
4 _____

Figure 1-6 in the textbook

Transverse Scanning Plane

4 sound wave approaches are possible
Anterior, Posterior,
Left lateral, or Right lateral

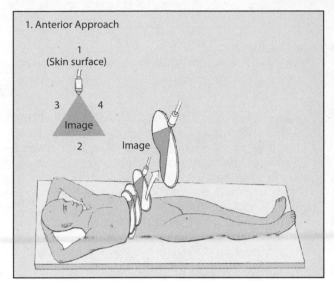

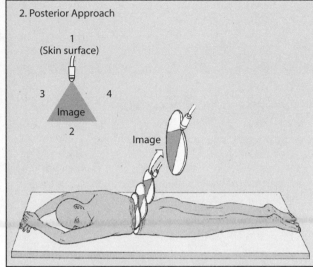

1 _____   1 _____

2 _____   2 _____

3 _____   3 _____

4 _____   4 _____

Figure 1-7, top, in the textbook

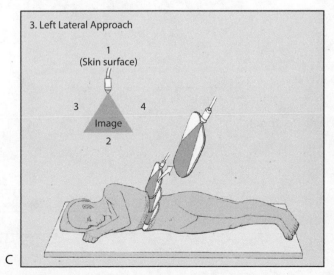

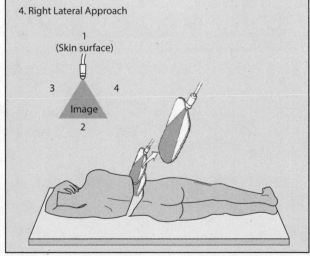

1 _____

2 _____

3 _____

4 _____

1 _____

2 _____

3 _____

4 _____

Figure 1-7, bottom, in the textbook

V. SYNTHESIS: DESCRIBING FINDINGS EXERCISE

1. Now it's your choice! For the following, you can label all of the sketches at once and then go back and label corresponding structures within each image with your lab partner, or work with an image and its accompanying sketch at the same time. Either way, the goal is to label all of the sketches correctly and carefully compare the sketch with the sonographic image.

2. Please review the section in your textbook titled How to Describe Ultrasound Findings. Use your textbook and write a description of the ultrasound findings below each image and accompanying sketch. Remember that you want to:
   - **differentiate** abnormal echo patterns from normal echo patterns,
   - **document** any differences in echo pattern appearance, and
   - **describe** any difference in echo pattern appearance using sonographic terminology.

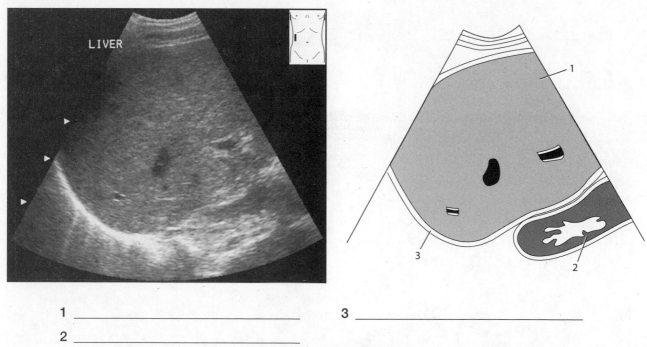

1 _____

2 _____

3 _____

Figure 1-9 in the textbook

Description:

_____

_____

_____

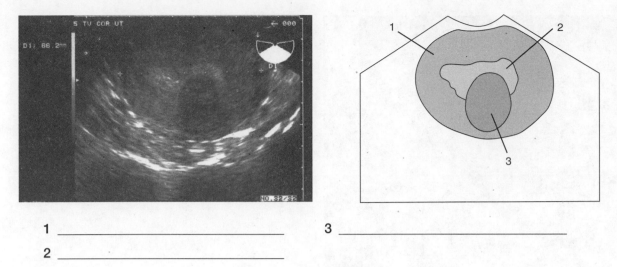

1 _____   3 _____

2 _____

Figure 1-10 in the textbook

Description:

_____

_____

_____

1 _____   3 _____

2 _____

Figure 1-11 in the textbook

Description:

_____

_____

_____

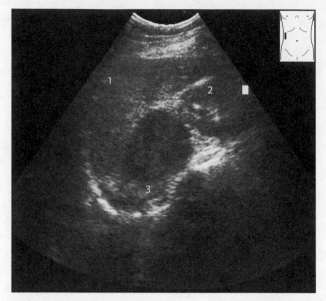

Figure 1-12 in the textbook

1 _____

2 _____

3 _____

Description:

_____

_____

_____

1 _____   3 _____

2 _____   4 _____

Figure 1-13 in the textbook

Description:

_____

_____

_____

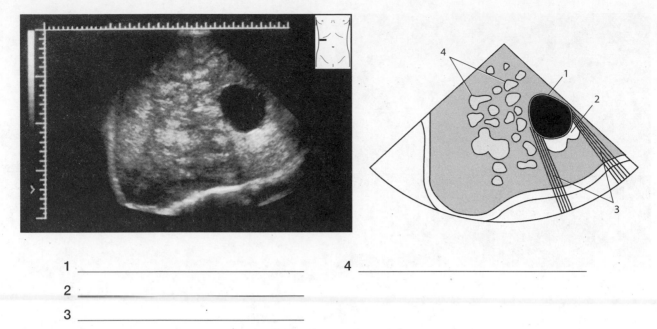

1 _____   4 _____

2 _____

3 _____

Figure 1-14 in the textbook

Description:

_____

_____

_____

1 _____   3 _____

2 _____   4 _____

Figure 1-15 in the textbook

Description:

_____

_____

_____

Chapter **1** **Before, During, and After the Ultrasound Exam**

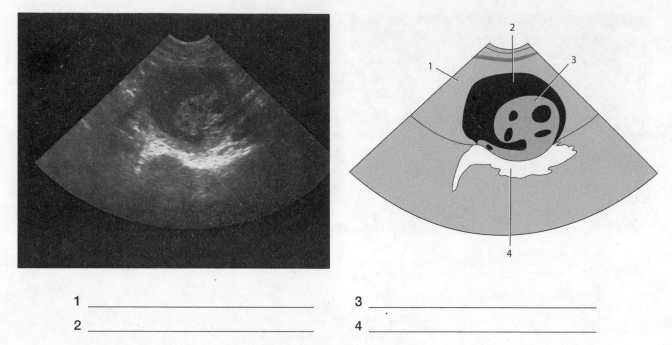

| 1 _____ | 3 _____ |
| 2 _____ | 4 _____ |

Figure 1-17 in the textbook

Description:

_____

_____

_____

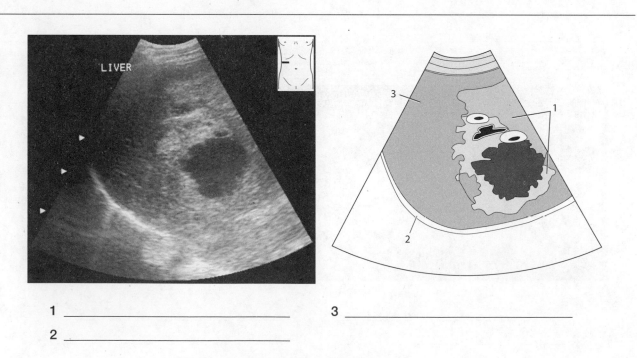

| 1 _____ | 3 _____ |
| 2 _____ | |

Figure 1-22 in the textbook

Description:

_____

_____

_____

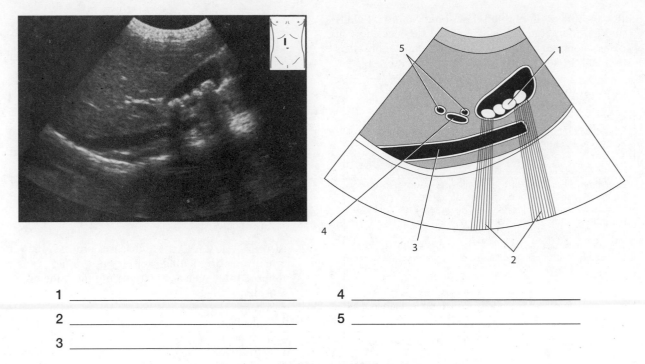

1 _____	4 _____
2 _____	5 _____
3 _____	

Figure 1-23 in the textbook

Description:

_____

_____

_____

1 _____	2 _____

Figure 1-24 in the textbook

Description:

_____

_____

_____

3. Review the examples of describing abnormal findings given in your textbook. What differences do you observe between the sonographer's technical observation and the sonologist's diagnosis in Figure 1-1?

FETAL AGE

DIAGNOSIS:

Findings compatible with complete spontaneous abortion, ectopic pregnancy, or very early intrauterine pregnancy.

COMMENT:

Real-time ultrasound of the pelvis was performed using transabdominal and endovaginal technique. No previous studies are available for review. The patient has a positive urine pregnancy test by history.

The uterus measures 10.2 x 4.2 x 5.0 cm. No intrauterine gestational sac is identified on transabdominal or endovaginal scan.

The left ovary is enlarged, measuring 4.2 x 2.9 x 3.6 cm. A cystic structure measuring less than 1 cm is seen in the left ovary.

The right ovary measures 2.6 x 1.1 x 2.8 cm. There are no right adnexal masses.

There is no free fluid in the cul de sac.

In light of the history of positive urine pregnancy test, the differential diagnosis for the above findings includes complete spontaneous abortion, ectopic pregnancy, or, less likely, very early intrauterine pregnancy. Correlation with serial beta-HCGs is advised.

Survey views of both kidneys reveal no hydronephrosis.

Figure 1-1 in the textbook

---

4. Working with your lab partner, demonstrate transducer placement for any of the images reviewed so far.

VI. CHAPTER EVALUATION EXERCISE

Use a fresh sheet of notebook paper. Based on your work with the chapter and its accompanying laboratory assignments, identify three concepts you believe are the most important. You may draw from any of the assignments you have already completed in the previous pages, including learning objectives, anatomy and physiology, images, or chapter subheadings. Include a detailed rationale in your answers.

Answer the questions below. Refer to page 369 for the answers.

Multiple Choice

1. The _____ is the point at which the sound beam is the narrowest and the resolution is the best.
   a. Doppler effect
   b. acoustic zone
   c. focal zone
   d. gray zone

2. _____ describes an irregular or mixed echo pattern on an ultrasound image.
   a. Doppler effect
   b. Heterogeneous
   c. Homogeneous
   d. Gray scale

3. _____ describes uniform or similar echo patterns on an ultrasound image.
   a. Doppler effect
   b. Heterogeneous
   c. Homogeneous
   d. Gray scale

4. A(n) _____ disease process may be visualized originating within an organ causing abnormalities such as external bulging of the organ's capsule.
   a. focal
   b. topical
   c. intra-organ
   d. extra-*organ*

Short Answer

5. List the three most important items from a patient's chart that sonographers need to review before performing an ultrasound exam.

6. Define what a sonographer can document within the parameters of a "technical observation."

7. Define what a sonographer can document within the parameters of a "technical observation" when there are abnormal findings on an exam.

8. Based on your work with the chapter and its accompanying laboratory assignments, identify three concepts you believe are the most important. You may draw from any of the assignments you have already completed in the previous pages, including learning objectives, anatomy and physiology, images, or chapter subheadings. Include a detailed rationale in your answers.

Completion

For the following questions, assign *CH* for clinical history, *TO* for technical observation, or *IR* for interpretive report.

8. Heterogeneous liver texture _____

9. Vomiting × 3 days _____

10. Right upper quadrant pain _____

11. Hepatomegaly _____

12. 4-cm aortic aneurysm _____

13. Portal hypertension _____

True/False

14. It is correct to say "The kidneys typically appear hypoechoic on a sonogram."

15. It is correct to say "The pancreas typically appears hyperechoic on a sonogram."

16. It is correct to say "Body structures are echogenic on a sonogram."

17. An abnormal mass within the body composed of one thing, tissue, is called a complex mass.

18. A complex mass is an abnormal mass within the body composed of both tissue and fluid.

19. An abnormal mass within the body composed only of fluid is described as a neoplasm.

Ultrasound Instrumentation: "Knobology," Imaging Processing, and Storage

2

I. MEMORIZATION EXERCISE

1. Write the key words in your notebook or on note cards. Write the words on one side of the notepaper and then write the definitions on the opposite side of the page or on the back of the paper. If using note cards, write the key word on the front and the definition on the back. *This step should be completed before the lab session begins.*

   Memorize the key word definitions silently for 5 minutes, then work with a lab partner and identify the words you still need help with. List the words here. Add additional rows if needed.

II. COMPREHENSION EXERCISE

1. Work with a lab partner to complete this exercise. You will need to write in your notebook. First, change each objective into a question.

   Example: "Explain why it is important to learn the 'knobology' of the ultrasound system" becomes "Why is it important to learn the 'knobology' of the ultrasound system?"

2. Next, write a short answer to the question just created.

   Example: "The sonographer has to know how each control affects the image, and how to work with all the controls to create the best image possible for the sonologist to use to render a diagnosis."

   Highlight or circle any part of your answers about which you are unsure, and check the answers in your textbook. If you are still unsure of the answers, put a question mark next to the answer(s) for the review session of the lab.

III. APPLICATION EXERCISE

1. Your instructor will distribute a section from an ultrasound systems manual for you and your partner to review. Can you identify the primary imaging controls, measurement controls, and additional controls presented in Chapter 2?

2. From memory, draw the control panel illustrated in question 1 above. Label the controls. Ask your partner to check your work and suggest additional controls that should be included.

IV. IMAGE ANALYSIS EXERCISE

Work on the following images with your lab partner. For each sonographic image, write an explanation in your notebook of the control settings used to render the image. How could the settings be improved? Refer to Chapter 2 in your textbook for guidance.

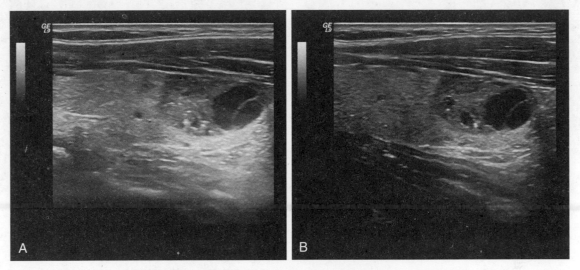

Figure 2-4A and B in the textbook

_____   _____

_____   _____

_____   _____

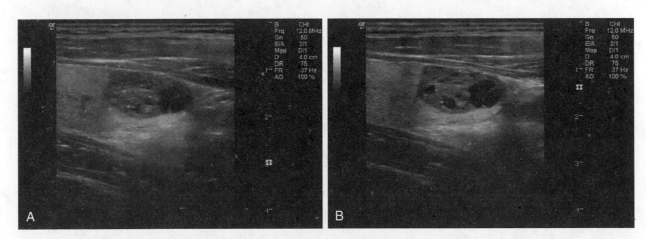

Figure 2-5A and B in the textbook

_____   _____

_____   _____

_____   _____

Chapter **2**   **Ultrasound Instrumentation: "Knobology," Imaging Processing, and Storage**

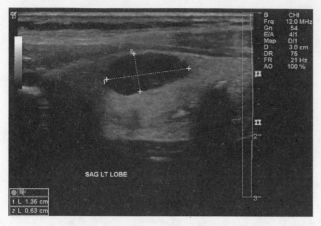

Figure 2-6 in the textbook

_____

_____

_____

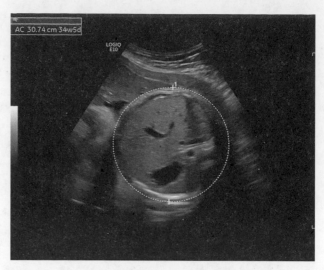

Figure 2-7 in the textbook

_____

_____

_____

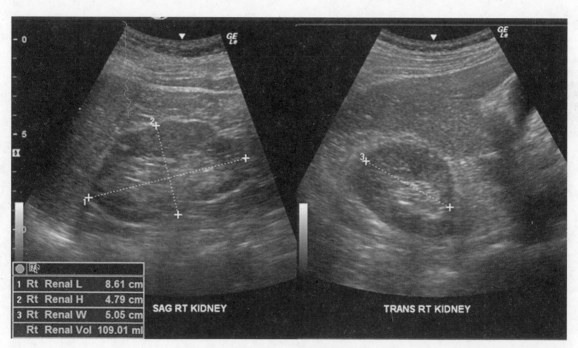

Figure 2-8 in the textbook

_____ _____

_____ _____

_____ _____

V. CHAPTER SUBHEADINGS EXERCISE

1. Convert each chapter subheading into a question. Briefly write the answer to each question in a short paragraph in your notebook. Exchange answers with your lab partner and check each other's work. Refer back to the textbook for further information and explanation.

2. What questions do you still have about the chapter? Write your questions in your notebook.

VI. CHAPTER EVALUATION EXERCISE

Use a fresh sheet of notebook paper. Based on your work with the chapter and its accompanying laboratory assignments, identify three concepts you believe are the most important. You may draw from any of the assignments you've already completed in the previous pages, including learning objectives, anatomy and physiology, images, or chapter subheadings. Include a detailed rationale in your answers.

Answer the questions below. Refer to page 369 for the answers.

Multiple Choice

1. Which function allows annotation to be entered on the screen?
   a. TGC Control
   b. Trace function
   c. Annotation On/Off
   d. Worklist

2. The reference manual for the ultrasound system can be accessed through which control?
   a. Clear control
   b. Primary imaging control menu
   c. Electronic program called "Worklist"
   d. Help menu

3. The "Worklist" electronic program allows the
   a. patient to update their medical record.
   b. sonographer to populate the patient information page.
   c. a & b
   d. None of the above

4. Primary imaging controls
   a. can be quickly learned by an experienced sonographer.
   b. indirectly impact imaging quality.

   c. a & b
   d. None of the above

5. Students need time to
   a. learn imaging controls.
   b. study the system manual.
   c. a & b
   d. None of the above

6. What is the function of the time-gain compensation (TGC) imaging control?
   a. It equalizes differences in received echo amplitudes.
   b. It activates the programmed storage device.
   c. It positions the focal zone to the desired scan depth.
   d. It suspends the image in real time.

7. Imaging frequency is higher for
   a. deeper structures.
   b. patients who have more body mass.
   c. superficial structures.
   d. All of the above

8. The trackball function
   a. controls the cursor on the screen.
   b. positions measurement cursors.
   c. changes the scan area.
   d. All of the above

9. Measurement keys and functions include
   a. imaging preset.
   b. image direction.
   c. trace.
   d. None of the above

10. The Body Pattern Control
    a. places cursors for distance measurements.
    b. is used to indicate patient positioning.
    c. changes imaging and trackball functions.
    d. can calculate volume measurements.

11. The sonographer uses the _____ to suspend images in real-time.
    a. Print/Store key
    b. Cine Loop control
    c. Freeze key
    d. Trackball

12. Small footprint transducers are listed below EXCEPT:
    a. 25 MHz
    b. 18 MHz
    c. 12 MHz
    d. 10 MHz

13. Transducers available for most units are listed below EXCEPT:
    a. Curved array
    b. Convex array
    c. Matrix array
    d. Concave array

General Patient Care 3

I. MEMORIZATION EXERCISE

1. Write the key words in your notebook or on note cards. Write the words on one side of the notepaper and then write the definitions on the opposite side of the page or on the back of the paper. If using note cards, write the key word on the front and the definition on the back. *This step should be completed before the lab session begins.*

   Memorize the key word definitions silently for 5 minutes, then work with a lab partner and identify the words you still need help with. List the words here. Add additional rows if needed.

II. COMPREHENSION EXERCISE

1. Work with a lab partner to complete this exercise. You will need to write in your notebook. First, change each objective into a question.

   Example: "Describe the sonographer's responsibilities regarding patient care" becomes "What are the sonographer's responsibilities regarding patient care?"

2. Next, write a short answer to the question just created.

   Example: "The sonographer should be aware of the institution's Standard Precautions and isolation policies and 'Code' procedures for incidences of heart failure. He or she should also check patient identification, assist patients who need help changing or positioning themselves, and instruct the patient in a slow, clear, and concise manner."

   Highlight or circle any part of your answers about which you are unsure, and check the answers in your textbook. If you are still unsure of the answers, put a question mark next to the answer(s) for the review session of the lab.

III. APPLICATION EXERCISE

1. Your instructor will provide mission statements from health care providers for you and your partner to review. Can you identify the patient care elements of the statement? In your opinion, does it clearly convey patient care standards to patients? How can the statement be "measured"? What types of outcomes would help measure the statement's validity?

2. Check your answers with your lab partner. Is there anything else you can add?

IV. CHAPTER SUBHEADINGS EXERCISE

1. Convert each chapter subheading into a question; for example, change "Interpersonal Skills" to, "What are the interpersonal skills used by sonographers in general patient care?" Write a brief answer to each question in a short paragraph in your notebook.

   Exchange answers with your lab partner and check each other's work. Refer back to the textbook for further information and explanation.

2. What questions do you still have about the chapter? Write your questions in your notebook.

VI. CHAPTER EVALUATION EXERCISE

Use a fresh sheet of notebook paper. Based on your work with the chapter and its accompanying laboratory assignments, identify three concepts you believe are the most important. You may draw from any of the assignments you've already completed in the previous pages, including learning objectives, anatomy and physiology, images, or chapter subheadings. Include a detailed rationale in your answers.

20

Answer the questions below. Refer to page 369 for the answers.

Multiple Choice

1. Patients may experience healthcare in which way?
   a. Confusing
   b. Emotionally draining
   c. Frightening
   d. All of the above

2. Patients deserve healthcare that is
   a. Respectful.
   b. Based on ability to pay.
   c. Considerate of their needs.
   d. A & C

3. During the sonography examination, who is responsible for the patient's well-being?
   a. referring physician
   b. Interpreting physician
   c. Sonographer
   d. Sonographer student

4. The sonographer can help the patient become more comfortable by doing the following EXCEPT
   a. Greet the patient with a smile.
   b. Speak very loudly to the patient – they may be hard of hearing.
   c. Make eye contact with the patient.
   d. Address them using first and last name.

5. Conversation with the patient should include
   a. Gently leading them back to the subject if needed.
   b. Using yes or no questions.
   c. Including medical acronyms so patient will understand better.
   d. Insisting that patients give detailed answers even when uncomfortable.

6. The ultrasound examination room should
   a. Be clean and clutter free.
   b. Have framed sonographer certificates that are easy to see.
   c. Include a well-stocked cabinet of supplies.
   d. All of the above

7. Sonographers should be aware of their institution's policies on
   a. Standard precautions and isolation.
   b. Code procedures.
   c. A & B
   d. None of the above

8. When explaining to an outpatient how to put on a hospital gown, which of the following is not acceptable?
   a. Keep the dressing area door or curtain fully open so you can make sure the patient is okay.
   b. Explain clothing that must be removed first.
   c. Ask if the patient needs assistance.
   d. Give adequate time to change.

9. Patient safety is increased when which of the following techniques are used?
   a. Set the brakes on the examination stretcher.
   b. Keep handled step stool nearby for use.
   c. Set brakes before helping patient out of wheelchair.
   d. All of the above

10. What information is not appropriate to tell a patient?
    a. The sonographer will provide the diagnosis after the procedure has ended.
    b. The room lights may be dimmed during the examination.
    c. The area to be examined will be exposed.
    d. A gel will be applied to the area to be examined.

11. Which is an invasive procedure?
    a. Applying gel to a patient's abdomen
    b. Performing an ultrasound-guided aspiration
    c. Checking the patient's chart to see whether they may have fluids
    d. Performing an ultrasound-guided physical examination

12. Aseptic technique is important for invasive procedures because it
    a. Creates a germ-free environment.
    b. Helps prevent pathogens from infecting the patient.
    c. Prevents the sonographer from getting sick.
    d. Keeps the procedure room clean and tidy.

13. Sonographers work under the delegated authority of the interpreting
    a. Nurse.
    b. Attorney.
    c. Physician.
    d. Technician.

Introduction to Ergonomics and Sonographer Safety   4

I. MEMORIZATION EXERCISE

1. Write the key words in your notebook or on note cards. Write the words on one side of the notepaper and then write the definitions on the opposite side of the page or on the back of the paper. If using note cards, write the key word on the front and the definition on the back. *This step should be completed before the lab session begins.*

   Memorize the key word definitions silently for 5 minutes, then work with a lab partner and identify the words you still need help with. List the words here. Add additional rows if needed.

II. COMPREHENSION EXERCISE

1. Work with a lab partner to complete this exercise. You will need to write in your notebook. First, change each objective into a question.

   Example: "List the types of patient injuries most likely to occur while scanning."

2. Next, write a short answer to the question just created.

   Example: "The types of injuries that can occur while scanning include bursitis, carpal tunnel syndrome, De Quervain's disease, tendon inflammation, plantar fasciitis, rotator cuff injury, and spinal degeneration."

   Highlight or circle any part of your answers about which you are unsure, and check the answers in your textbook. If you are still unsure of the answers, put a question mark next to the answer(s) for the review session of the lab.

III. APPLICATION EXERCISE

1. For each workplace activity or condition listed below, discuss proactive approaches to reduce work-related musculoskeletal disorders and musculoskeletal injuries:
   - Workspace design
   - Infrequent breaks or rest periods
   - Incentives for overtime and being on-call
   - Delayed injury reporting
   - Improper cable management
   - Improper sitting height of chair
   - Monitor too low, causing flexion of the neck
   - "Pinch grip" of the transducer
   - Air quality factors such as heat, cold, humidity
   - Poor posture
   - Increase in the number of portable exams
   - Sustained shoulder abduction
   - Aging workforce
   - Staffing shortages
   - Higher workloads due to advancement in technology

2. What are the most important strategies sonographers can use to reduce injuries? Provide a rationale for your answers.

IV. CHAPTER SUBHEADINGS EXERCISE

1. Convert each chapter subheading into a question; for example, change "Work-Related Musculoskeletal Disorders" to "What are the work-related musculoskeletal disorders?" Write a brief answer to each question in a short paragraph in your notebook.

   Exchange answers with your lab partner and check each other's work. Refer back to the textbook for further information and explanation.

2. What questions do you still have about the chapter? Write your questions in your notebook.

V. CHAPTER EVALUATION EXERCISE

Use a fresh sheet of notebook paper. Based on your work with the chapter and its accompanying laboratory assignments, identify three concepts you believe are the most important. You may draw from any of the assignments you've already completed in the previous pages, including learning objectives, anatomy and physiology, images, or chapter subheadings. Include a detailed rationale in your answers.

Answer the questions below. Refer to page 369 for the answers.

Multiple Choice

1. What percentage of sonographers retires early because of pain due to WRMSD?
   a. 100%
   b. 20%
   c. 50%
   d. 90%

2. The patient should be placed no more than_____% away to avoid reaching to scan.
   a. 10
   b. 50
   c. 90
   d. 30

3. Which of the following equipment design issues would significantly contribute to wrist and hand strain for sonographers?
   a. Transducer weight
   b. Ultrasound gel
   c. Cable support brace
   d. Adjustable chair

4. Which of the following would benefit someone with WRMSD?
   a. Rest
   b. Good posture
   c. Stretching exercises
   d. All of the above

5. Which of the following would not aggravate musculoskeletal symptoms?
   a. Sustained twisting of the neck and trunk
   b. Sustained neutral wrist position
   c. Sustained shoulder abduction
   d. Sustained transducer pressure

Completion

6. A _____ _____ is a device used to support the scanning arm of the transducer.

7. _____ _____ are similar movements that may be required to perform a task.

8. _____ relates to how much pressure is applied by one object (transducer) to the surface of another object (the patient).

9. _____ is when part of the body (such as the arm) is moved away from the midline.

10. A _____ _____ _____ is a device which is placed on the arm to hold the cord of a transducer in place while scanning.

11. The knowledge of_____ can create a safe scanning environment for the sonographer, vascular technologist, and sonologist.

Short Answer

12. Explain the 20-20-20 rule that sonographers should practice during the scan time.

13. Name 3 workplace activities that can cause WRMSD injuries.

Interdependent Body Systems 5

I. MEMORIZATION EXERCISE

1. Write the key words in your notebook or on note cards. Write the words on one side of the notepaper and then write the definitions on the opposite side of the page or on the back of the paper. If using note cards, write the key word on the front and the definition on the back. *This step should be completed before the lab session begins*.

    Memorize the key word definitions silently for 5 minutes, then work with a lab partner and identify the words you still need help with. List the words here. Add additional rows if needed.

II. COMPREHENSION EXERCISE

1. Work with a lab partner to complete this exercise. You will need to write in your notebook. Select one of the body systems discussed in the chapter and describe its function(s).

    Highlight or circle any part of your answers about which you are unsure, and check the answers in your textbook. If you are still unsure of the answers, put a question mark next to the answer(s) for the review session of the lab.

III. ANATOMY APPLICATION EXERCISE

1. After reviewing the illustrations of these systems in your textbook, draw the major components of the endocrine, circulatory, musculoskeletal, reproductive, urinary, digestive, and respiratory systems in your notebook. (Do this with the textbook closed.) How many structures were you able to include in your drawing? Review your diagrams with your partner. What did you miss?

2. Check your drawing using the sketches in your textbook and complete any structures missing from your drawing.

3. Below your drawing, write two or three summary sentences for each system. Ask your lab partner to check your work. Now check your work against the explanations in the textbook. What else can you add to your description?

IV. CHAPTER SUBHEADINGS EXERCISE

1. Convert each chapter subheading into a question; for example, change "Digestive System" to "What is the digestive system and how does it relate to other body systems?" Write a brief answer to each question in a short paragraph in your notebook. Exchange answers with your lab partner and check each other's work. Refer back to the textbook for further information and explanation.

2. What questions do you still have about the chapter? Write your questions in your notebook.

V. CHAPTER EVALUATION EXERCISE

Use a fresh sheet of notebook paper. Based on your work with the chapter and its accompanying laboratory assignments, identify three concepts you believe are the most important. You may draw from any of the assignments you've already completed in the previous pages, including learning objectives, anatomy and physiology, images, or chapter subheadings. Include a detailed rationale in your answers.

Answer the questions below. Refer to page 369 for the answers.

Completion

1. _____ transfer instructions from one set of cells to another.

2. The _____ is a collection of glands that secrete hormones directly into the bloodstream to arrive at _____.

3. The _____ is the "master gland" of the endocrine system and is also known as the _____.

4. The _____ sits in the sella turcica.

5. The _____ is connected to the _____ by a stalk, through which it receives instructions on how to regulate hormonal activity.

6. _____ is a wormlike motion that moves contents along the large bowel.

7. The _____ phase of the heart is called diastole.

8. The _____ phase of the heart is called systole.

9. One of the main functions of the _____ is collection and transportation of excess fluids from interstitial spaces of the body back into veins in the bloodstream.

10. At the end of each skeletal muscle, the collagen fibers come together to form a bundle known as a _____.

11. Tendons attach muscles to _____.

12. Bones are connected to each other by _____.

13. _____ occurs within the marrow of bones.

Anatomy Layering and Sectional Anatomy 6

I. MEMORIZATION EXERCISE

1. Write the key words in your notebook or on note cards. Write the words on one side of the notepaper and then write the definitions on the opposite side of the page or on the back of the paper. If using note cards, write the key word on the front and the definition on the back. *This step should be completed before the lab session begins.*

   Memorize the key word definitions silently for 5 minutes and then work with a lab partner and identify the words you still need help with. List the words here. Add rows if needed.

II. COMPREHENSION EXERCISE

1. Work with a lab partner to complete this exercise. You will need to write in your notebook. First, change each objective into a question.

   Example: "Explain the importance of using two different scanning planes" becomes "Why is it important to use two different scanning planes?"

2. Next, write a short answer to the question just created.

   Example: "Multiple scanning planes are used in ultrasound imaging because single plane views do not provide enough confirmation to make definitive judgments."

   Highlight or circle any part of your answers about which you are unsure, and check the answers in your textbook. If you are still unsure of the answers, put a question mark next to the answer(s) for the review session of the lab.

III. ANATOMY APPLICATION EXERCISE

1. Using clay or any other product that is easy to shape, re-create Figures 6-4 to 6-12 (in the textbook), the abdominal layers, and Figures 6-13 to 6-17 (in the textbook), the pelvic layers, building the anatomy in layers from posterior (back) to anterior (front). Label each structure, taping the label to toothpicks, before inserting into the structure. When the layers are complete, use a knife to cut out various axial and longitudinal sections; identify the anatomy in these cross-sections.

IV. STRUCTURAL ORIENTATION EXERCISE

1. On the following page, identify each numbered structure from Table 6-2 (in the textbook) and its orientation (or lie) within the body.

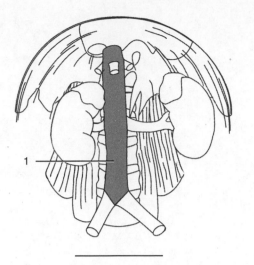

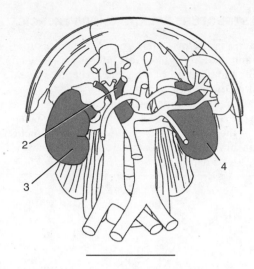

1 _____

2 _____

3 _____

4 _____

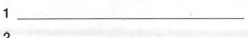

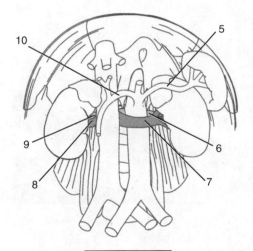

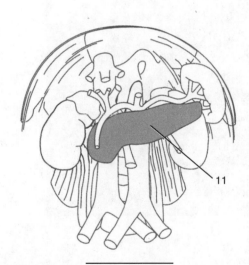

(the lateral end of the pancreas is slightly more
superior than the medial end)

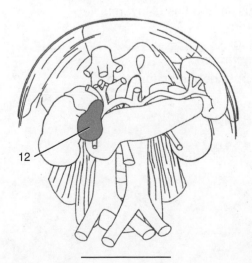

5 _____

6 _____

7 _____

8 _____

9 _____

10 _____

11 _____

12 _____

Table 6-2 in the textbook

Chapter **6** **Anatomy Layering and Sectional Anatomy**

V. BODY STRUCTURE RELATIONSHIPS EXERCISE

Use directional terms—anterior, posterior, superior, inferior, and medial, right or left lateral—as they apply to describe the location of adjacent structures to a designated area of interest.

1. Transabdominal sagittal scanning plane image taken just to the left of the midline of the body. The pancreas body is the area of interest. Identify the directional relationship of the adjacent anatomy.

Example: Liver: anterior.

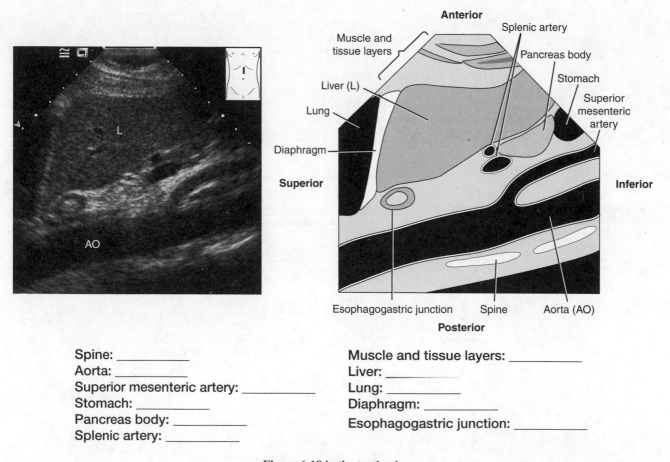

Spine: _____
Aorta: _____
Superior mesenteric artery: _____
Stomach: _____
Pancreas body: _____
Splenic artery: _____

Muscle and tissue layers: _____
Liver: _____
Lung: _____
Diaphragm: _____
Esophagogastric junction: _____

Figure 6-18 in the textbook

2. Transabdominal coronal scanning plane image from a left lateral approach. The superior pole of the left kidney is the area of interest. Identify the directional relationship of the adjacent anatomy.

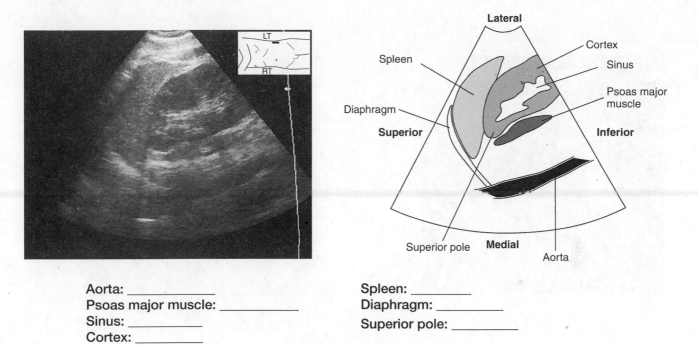

Aorta: _____
Psoas major muscle: _____
Sinus: _____
Cortex: _____

Spleen: _____
Diaphragm: _____
Superior pole: _____

Figure 6-19 in the textbook

3. Transabdominal transverse scanning plane image taken at the level of the midepigastrium. The pancreas neck is the area of interest. Identify the directional relationship of the adjacent anatomy.

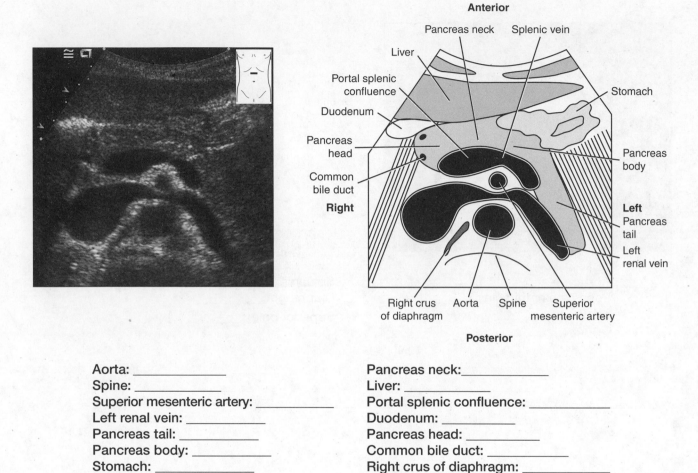

Aorta: _____
Spine: _____
Superior mesenteric artery: _____
Left renal vein: _____
Pancreas tail: _____
Pancreas body: _____
Stomach: _____
Splenic vein: _____

Pancreas neck:_____
Liver: _____
Portal splenic confluence: _____
Duodenum: _____
Pancreas head: _____
Common bile duct: _____
Right crus of diaphragm: _____

Figure 6-20 in the textbook

VI. COMPARING ULTRASOUND IMAGE SECTIONS WITH CORRESPONDING GROSS ANATOMY LAYERS EXERCISE

Identify the labeled anatomy in the image on the corresponding gross anatomy layers.

1. Transabdominal sagittal scanning plane image taken just to the right of the midline of the body (represented by the solid line on the layering illustrations).

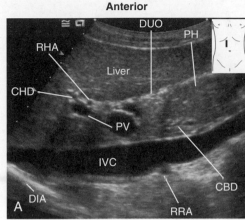

Figure 6-21A in the textbook DIA (diaphragm), RRA (right renal artery), IVC (inferior vena cava), PV (portal vein), CBD (common bile duct), PH (pancreas head), CHD (common hepatic duct), RHA (right hepatic artery), DUO (duodenum)

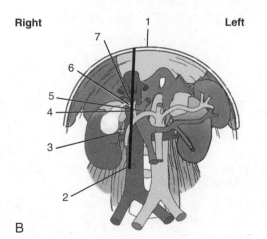

1 _____

2 _____

3 _____

4 _____

5 _____

6 _____

7 _____

Figure 6-21B in the textbook

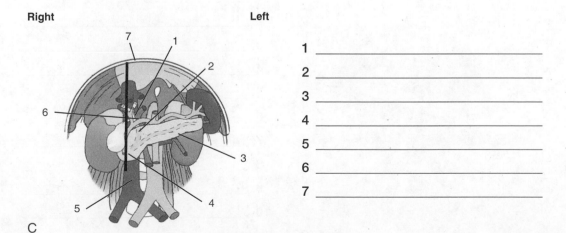

1 _____

2 _____

3 _____

4 _____

5 _____

6 _____

7 _____

Figure 6-21C in the textbook

Chapter **6** Anatomy Layering and Sectional Anatomy

2. Transabdominal transverse scanning plane image of the mid to lower epigastrium (represented by the dotted line on the layering illustrations).

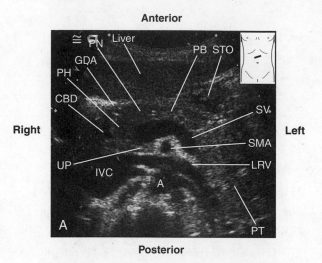

Figure 6-22A in the textbook A (aorta), IVC (inferior vena cava), LRV (left renal vein), SMA (superior mesenteric artery), UP (uncinate process of the pancreas), PT (pancreas tail), SV (splenic vein), SMA (superior mesenteric artery), PH (pancreas head), CBD (common bile duct), PN (pancreas neck), GDA (gastroduodenal artery), PB (pancreas body), STO (stomach)

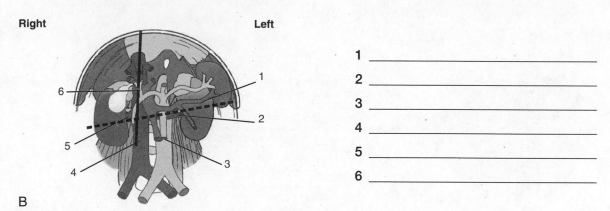

1 _____
2 _____
3 _____
4 _____
5 _____
6 _____

Figure 6-22B in the textbook

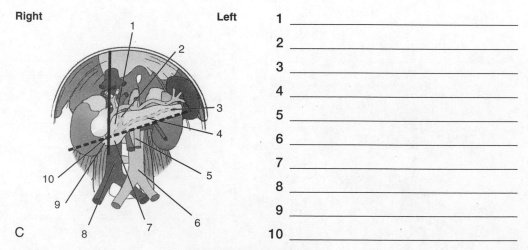

1 _____
2 _____
3 _____
4 _____
5 _____
6 _____
7 _____
8 _____
9 _____
10 _____

Figure 6-22C in the textbook

Chapter **6** Anatomy Layering and Sectional Anatomy

VII. ANATOMY SYNTHESIS EXERCISE: ANATOMY LAYERS AND ILLUSTRATIONS

Work on the following with your lab partner. Label all abdominal sketches at once and then go back and work with each figure with your lab partner to check your answers. The goal is to label all of the sketches correctly.

1.

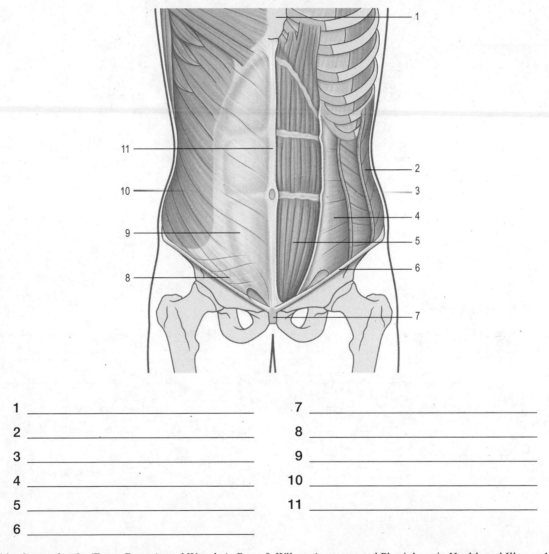

1	_____	7	_____
2	_____	8	_____
3	_____	9	_____
4	_____	10	_____
5	_____	11	_____
6	_____		

Figure 6-4 in the textbook (From Grant A. and Waugh A. Ross & Wilson Anatomy and Physiology in Health and Illness. 13th ed., Edinburgh, 2018, Elsevier.)

2.

Right   **Left**

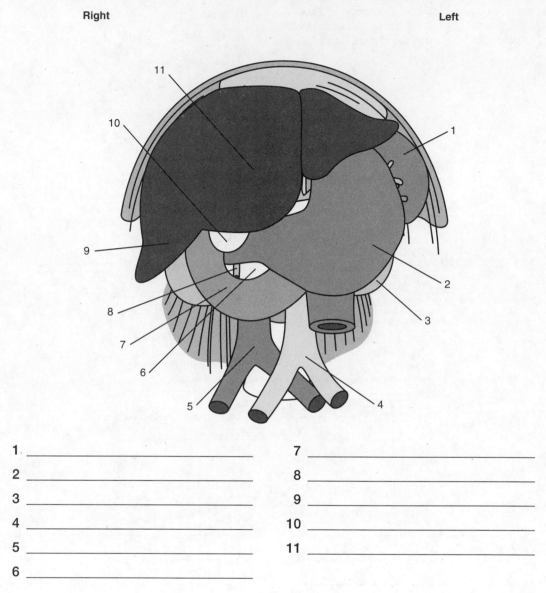

1. _____   7. _____
2. _____   8. _____
3. _____   9. _____
4. _____   10. _____
5. _____   11. _____
6. _____

Figure 6-5 in the textbook

3.

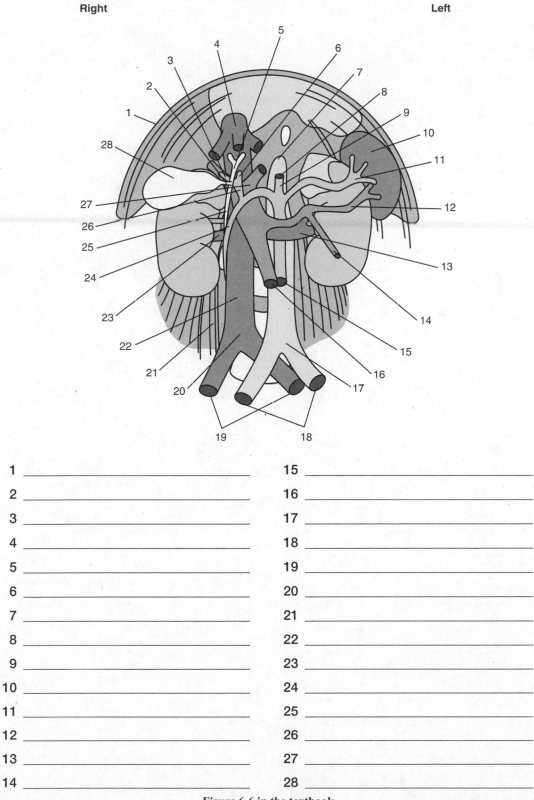

Right   **Left**

Figure 6-6 in the textbook

1	_____	15	_____
2	_____	16	_____
3	_____	17	_____
4	_____	18	_____
5	_____	19	_____
6	_____	20	_____
7	_____	21	_____
8	_____	22	_____
9	_____	23	_____
10	_____	24	_____
11	_____	25	_____
12	_____	26	_____
13	_____	27	_____
14	_____	28	_____

4.

Figure 6-7 in the textbook

1 _____	10 _____
2 _____	11 _____
3 _____	12 _____
4 _____	13 _____
5 _____	14 _____
6 _____	15 _____
7 _____	16 _____
8 _____	17 _____
9 _____	18 _____

5.

Right   **Left**

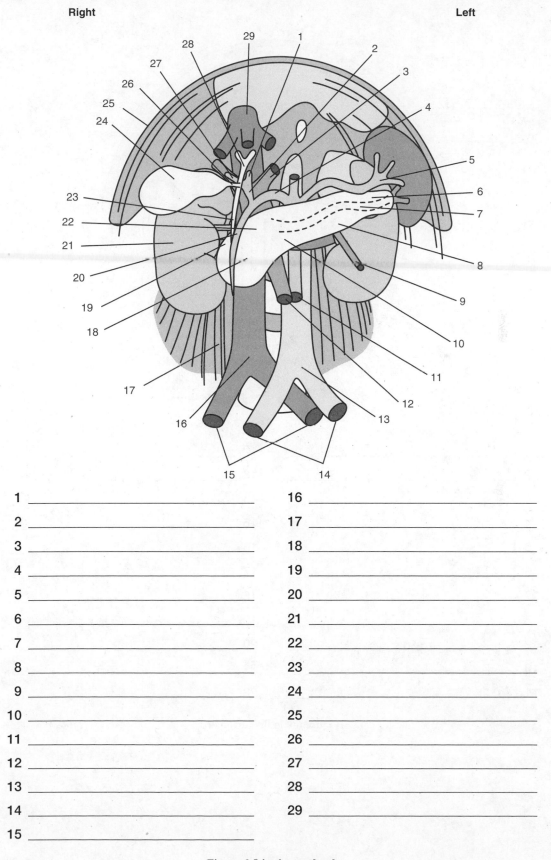

1	_____	16	_____
2	_____	17	_____
3	_____	18	_____
4	_____	19	_____
5	_____	20	_____
6	_____	21	_____
7	_____	22	_____
8	_____	23	_____
9	_____	24	_____
10	_____	25	_____
11	_____	26	_____
12	_____	27	_____
13	_____	28	_____
14	_____	29	_____
15	_____		

Figure 6-8 in the textbook

Chapter **6**   **Anatomy Layering and Sectional Anatomy**

6.

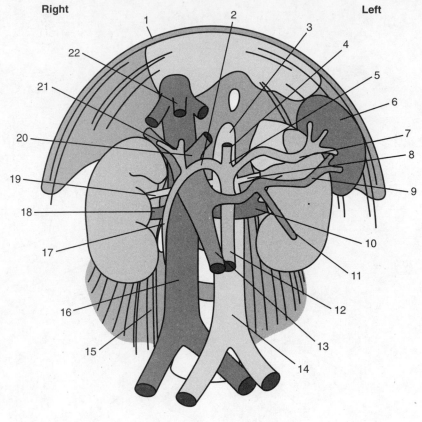

Right **Left**

1 _____   12 _____
2 _____   13 _____
3 _____   14 _____
4 _____   15 _____
5 _____   16 _____
6 _____   17 _____
7 _____   18 _____
8 _____   19 _____
9 _____   20 _____
10 _____   21 _____
11 _____   22 _____

Figure 6-9 in the textbook

7.

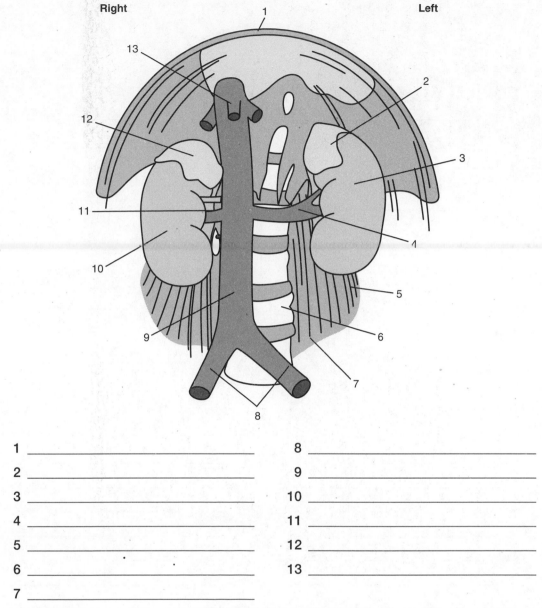

Right   Left

1	_____	8	_____
2	_____	9	_____
3	_____	10	_____
4	_____	11	_____
5	_____	12	_____
6	_____	13	_____
7	_____		

Figure 6-10 in the textbook

8.

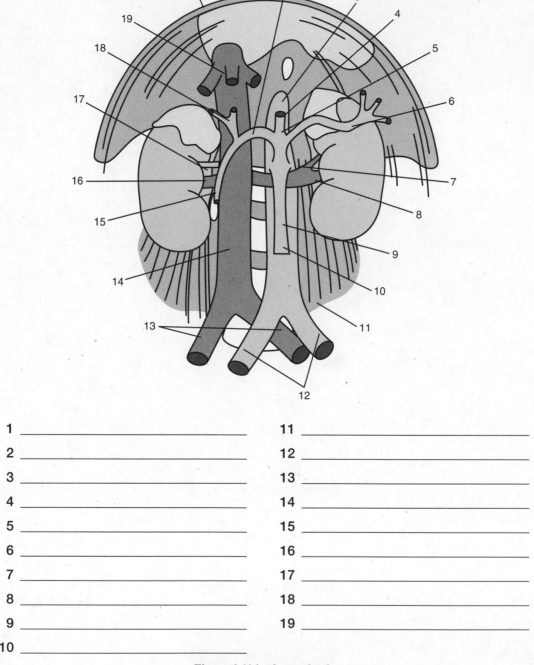

Right   Left

Figure 6-11 in the textbook

1	_____	11	_____
2	_____	12	_____
3	_____	13	_____
4	_____	14	_____
5	_____	15	_____
6	_____	16	_____
7	_____	17	_____
8	_____	18	_____
9	_____	19	_____
10	_____		

9.

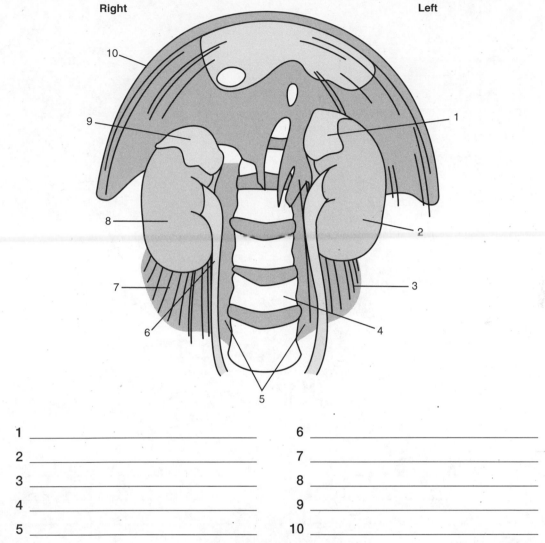

Right   Left

1	_____	6	_____
2	_____	7	_____
3	_____	8	_____
4	_____	9	_____
5	_____	10	_____

Figure 6-12 in the textbook

Chapter **6** **Anatomy Layering and Sectional Anatomy**

Label all of the pelvic images (1–6) at once and then go back and work with each figure with your lab partner. The goal is to label all of the sketches correctly.

1.

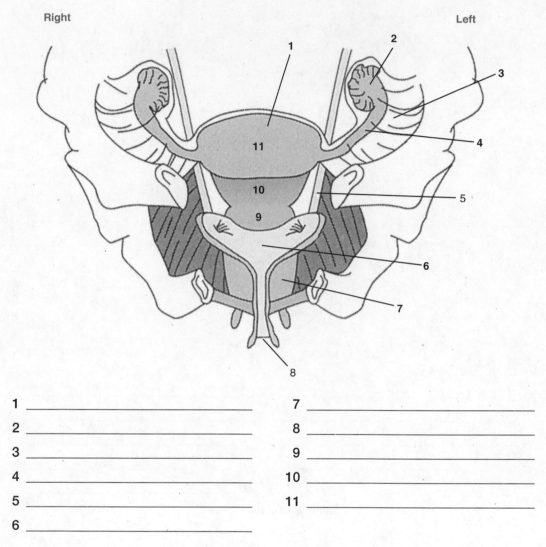

Right   Left

1	_____	7	_____
2	_____	8	_____
3	_____	9	_____
4	_____	10	_____
5	_____	11	_____
6	_____		

Figure 6-13 in the textbook

2.

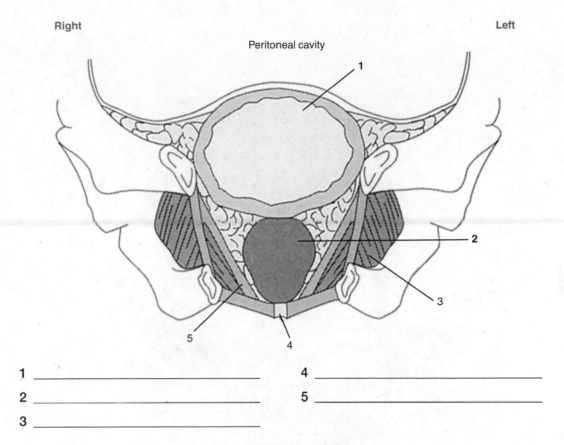

Right   Left

Peritoneal cavity

1 _____   4 _____

2 _____   5 _____

3 _____

Figure 6-14 in the textbook

Chapter **6**   **Anatomy Layering and Sectional Anatomy**

3.

Right

Left

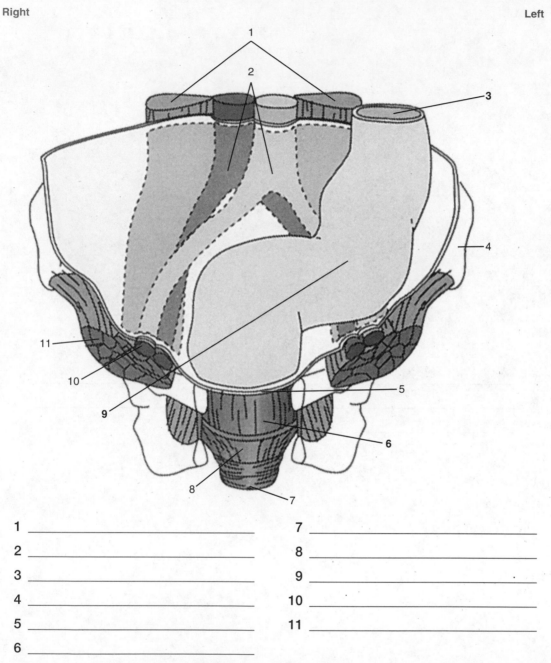

1 _____   7 _____
2 _____   8 _____
3 _____   9 _____
4 _____   10 _____
5 _____   11 _____
6 _____

Figure 6-15 in the textbook

Chapter **6**   **Anatomy Layering and Sectional Anatomy**

4.

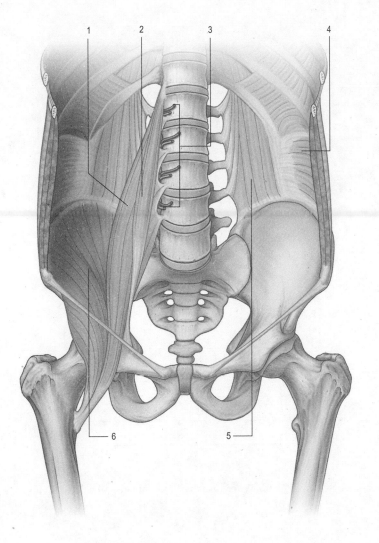

1 _____

2 _____

3 _____

4 _____

5 _____

6 _____

Figure 6-16 in the textbook (From Standring S. Gray's Anatomy. 41st ed., London, 2016, Elsevier.)

5.

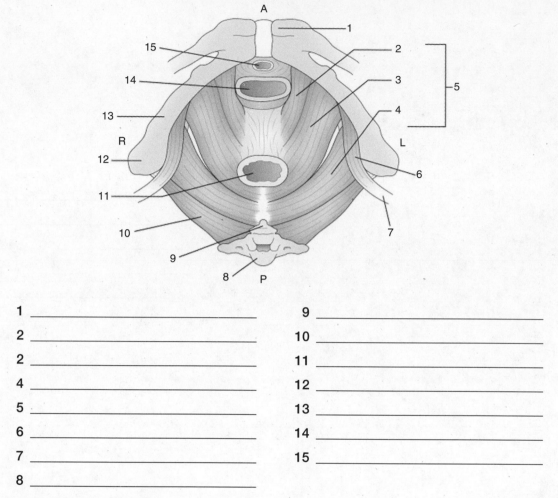

Figure 6-17 in the textbook (From Kelley L.L. and Petersen C.M. Sectional Anatomy for Imaging Professionals. 4th ed., St. Louis, 2018, Elsevier.)

1	_____	9	_____
2	_____	10	_____
2	_____	11	_____
4	_____	12	_____
5	_____	13	_____
6	_____	14	_____
7	_____	15	_____
8	_____		

VIII. CHAPTER EVALUATION EXERCISE

Use a fresh sheet of notebook paper. Based on your work with the chapter and its accompanying laboratory assignments, identify three concepts you believe are most important. You may draw from any of the assignments you have already completed in the previous pages, including learning objectives, anatomy and physiology, images, or chapter subheadings. Include a detailed rationale in your answers.

Answer to the questions below. Refer to page 369 for the answers.

Label the following body structures as intraperitoneal (P) or retroperitoneal (R) or both (B):

1. Right kidney _____

2. Left kidney _____

3. Stomach _____

4. Liver _____

5. Pancreas _____

6. Ovaries _____

7. Prostate gland _____

8. Ascending colon _____

9. Descending colon _____

10. Duodenum _____

11. Spleen _____

12. Gallbladder _____

13. The part of the axial skeleton which links the lower extremities to the rest of the body through the lumbosacral spine is called the
    a. coccyx.
    b. hipbones.
    c. pelvis.
    d. vertebral column.

14. Which of the following would be normally considered to have a vertical oblique orientation or lie within the human body?
    a. Common bile duct
    b. Thyroid isthmus
    c. Right renal artery
    d. Pancreas

15. Which of the following would be normally considered to have a horizontal oblique orientation or lie within the human body?
    a. Common bile duct
    b. Thyroid isthmus
    c. Right renal artery
    d. Pancreas

16. The plane which divides the body into right and left sections parallel to the long axis of the midline is known as the _____ plane.
    a. transverse
    b. sagittal
    c. coronal
    d. axial

17. The plane which divides the body into anterior and posterior sections perpendicular to the longitudinal plane and parallel to the long axis of the body from the midaxillary line is better known as the _____ plane.
    a. transverse
    b. sagittal
    c. coronal
    d. axial

18. In a *transverse scanning plane* image, the target organ or area of interest is always related to a structure immediately
    a. anterior, posterior, inferior or superior to it.
    b. right or left lateral, medial, superior or inferior to it.
    c. anterior, posterior, medial, right or left lateral to it.
    d. superior or inferior, coronal or medial to it.

19. Multiple scanning planes are utilized in ultrasound imaging because
    a. they generate volume measurements, a complete assessment and the findings are thus considered confirmed and reliable.
    b. perpendicular imaging planes are more reliable than parallel plane imaging of structures.
    c. something imaged in a single plane cannot be considered reliable unless a volume measurement can be generated from the same plane.
    d. they provide confirmation of refracted echoes that are not returned from a single plane imaged.

20. Which of the following vessels originates from the left upper quadrant and courses horizontally and medial toward the midline before terminating posterior to the neck of the pancreas?
    a. Portal vein
    b. Splenic vein
    c. Gastroduodenal artery
    d. Left gastric artery

21. Which of the following structures is not a part of the biliary tract?
    a. Right hepatic duct
    b. Common bile duct
    c. Duct of Wirsung
    d. Cystic duct

22. Each of the following marks a segment of the large bowel EXCEPT the
    a. cecum.
    b. splenic flexure.
    c. jejunum.
    d. rectum.

Embryology 7

I. MEMORIZATION EXERCISE

1. Write the key words in your notebook or on note cards. Write the words on one side of the notepaper and then write the definitions on the opposite side of the page or on the back of the paper. If using note cards, write the key word on the front and the definition on the back. *This step should be completed before the lab session begins.*

   Memorize the key word definitions silently for 5 minutes, then work with a lab partner and identify the words you still need help with. List the words here. Add additional rows if needed.

II. COMPREHENSION EXERCISE

1. Work with a lab partner to complete this exercise. You will need to write in your notebook. First, change each objective into a question.

   Example: "Describe the three layers of the embryo and the organs formed from each layer" becomes "What are the three layers of the embryo and which organs are formed from each layer?"

2. Next, write a short answer to the question just created.

   Example: "The embryo consists of three layers; the most external is the ectoderm (brain and spinal cord); the middle mesoderm (heart, circulatory, kidneys, and reproductive systems); and the inner layer, endoderm (lungs, intestines, and urinary bladder)."

   Highlight or circle any part of your answers about which you are unsure, and check the answers in your textbook. If you are still unsure of the answers, put a question mark next to the answer(s) for the review session of the lab.

III. APPLICATION OF ANATOMY AND PHYSIOLOGY EXERCISE

1. Layers: Label the figure. Write a brief description of the function of the layers described in the figure.

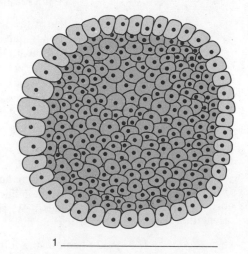

1 _____

Description:

_____

_____

_____

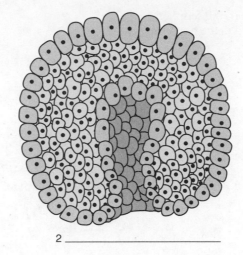

2 _____

Description:

_____
_____
_____

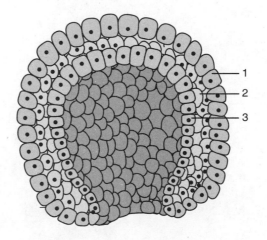

1 _____   3 _____
2 _____

Figure 7-1 in the textbook

Description:

_____
_____
_____

2. Vessels: Label the figure. Write a brief description of the function of the vessels described in the figure.

Superior   Inferior

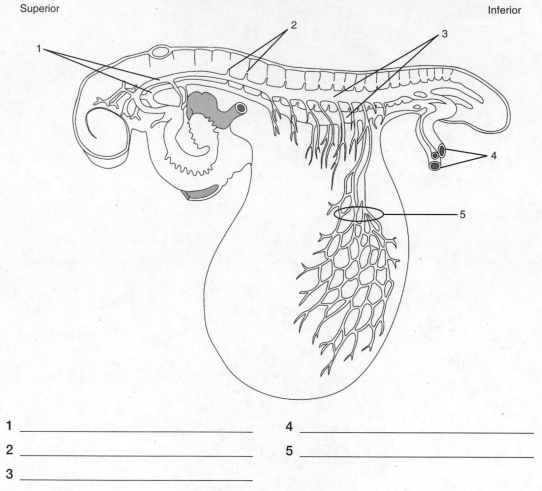

1 _____   4 _____

2 _____   5 _____

3 _____

Figure 7-2 in the textbook

Description:

_____

_____

_____

3. Organs: Label the figures. Write a brief description of the function of each organ represented in the figures.

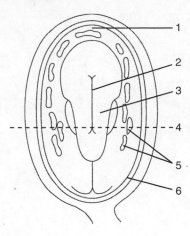

1
2
3
4
5
6

Description:

_____

_____

_____

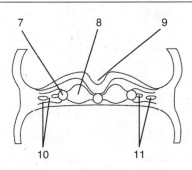

7   8   9

10   11

Description:

_____

_____

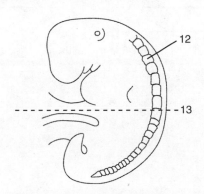

12

13

Description:

_____

_____

_____

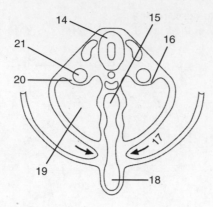

Description:

_____

_____

_____

1 _____   12 _____

2 _____   13 _____

3 _____   14 _____

4 _____   15 _____

5 _____   16 _____

6 _____   17 _____

7 _____   18 _____

8 _____   19 _____

9 _____   20 _____

10 _____   21 _____

11 _____

Figure 7-3 in the textbook

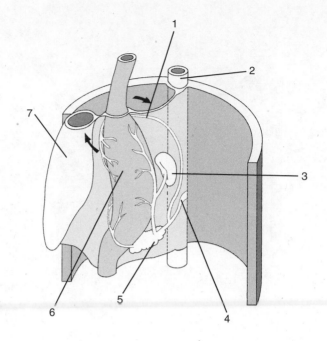

Description:

_____

_____

_____

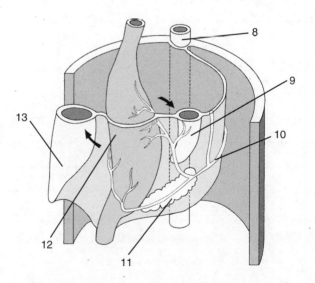

Description:

_____

_____

_____

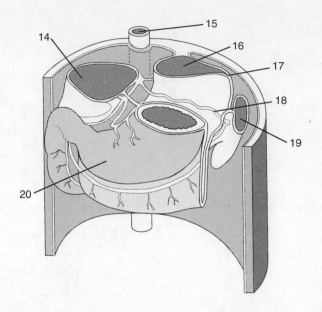

Description:

_____

_____

_____

1 _____   11 _____

2 _____   12 _____

3 _____   13 _____

4 _____   14 _____

5 _____   15 _____

6 _____   16 _____

7 _____   17 _____

8 _____   18 _____

9 _____   19 _____

10 _____   20 _____

Figure 7-4 in the textbook

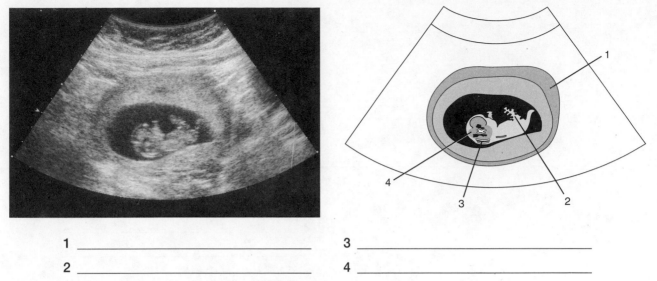

Figure 7-5 in the textbook

1 _____   3 _____

2 _____   4 _____

Description:

_____

_____

_____

1 **Herniation**

2 Umbilicus / **Counterclockwise rotation**

3 **Small bowel**

4 Colon / **Affixed framework**

1 _____   3 _____

2 _____   4 _____

Figure 7-6 in the textbook

Description:

_____

_____

_____

55

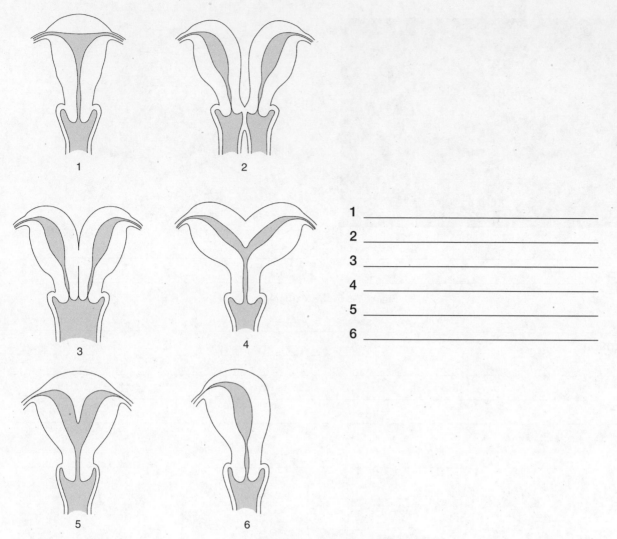

1 _____
2 _____
3 _____
4 _____
5 _____
6 _____

Figure 7-12 in the textbook

Description:

_____

_____

_____

4. Brain and neck: Label the figure. Write a brief description of the function of each organ represented in the figure.

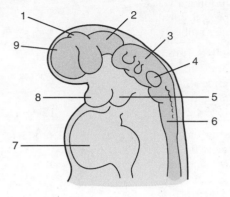

Figure 7-19 in the textbook

1 _____
2 _____
3 _____
4 _____
5 _____
6 _____
7 _____
8 _____
9 _____

Description:

_____

_____

_____

IV. CHAPTER SUBHEADINGS EXERCISE

1. Convert each chapter subheading into a question; for example, change "Liver Development" to "What is the embryological development of the liver?" Briefly answer each question in a short paragraph in your notebook. Exchange answers with your lab partner and check each other's work. Refer back to the textbook for further information and explanation.
2. What questions do you still have about the chapter? Write your questions in your notebook.

V. CHAPTER EVALUATION EXERCISE

Use a fresh sheet of notebook paper. Based on your work with the chapter and its accompanying laboratory assignments, identify three concepts you believe are the most important. You may draw from any of the assignments you've already completed in the previous pages, including learning objectives, anatomy and physiology, images, or chapter subheadings. Include a detailed rationale in your answers.

Answer the questions below. Refer to page 370 for the answers.

Multiple Choice

1. The diencaphalon is composed of
   a. skin cells.
   b. the genital organs.
   c. the thalamus and hypothalamus.
   d. cardiac tissue.

2. The Mullerian ducts develop alongside the mesonephros into the
   a. testes.
   b. rectum.
   c. prostate.
   d. female genital tract.

3. After birth, the umbilical vein degenerates into the
   a. ductus venosus.
   b. ligamentum teres.
   c. diencephalon.
   d. ectoderm.

4. Wolffian ducts are paramesonephric ducts that develop into the
   a. male genital tract.
   b. telencephalon.
   c. tailgut.
   d. umbilical arteries.

5. All of the following are true about Carnegie stages EXCEPT:
   a. They are used to describe embryologic maturity.
   b. They are based on physical characteristics.
   c. They are numbered 1 to 23.
   d. Stage 1 is the most advanced and stage 23 is the least advanced.

6. Deoxygenated blood is returned to the placenta by the
   a. umbilical arteries.
   b. umbilical veins.
   c. prosencephalon.
   d. heart tubes.

7. The liver is formed from the
   a. hindgut.
   b. midgut.
   c. tailgut.
   d. foregut.

8. During embryonic life blood cell production takes place in the
   a. mesonephros.
   b. spleen.
   c. pancreas.
   d. liver.

9. The most appropriate sequence of neural development is
   a. telencephalon, prosencephalon, diencephalon, neural tube.
   b. neural tube, neurons, thalamus.
   c. neural tube, prosencephalon, diencephalon, telencephalon.
   d. telencephalon, diencephalon.

10. After birth, the ductus venosus becomes the
    a. forebrain.
    b. heart.
    c. ligamentum venosum.
    d. splenic ridge.

8 Introduction to Laboratory Values

I. MEMORIZATION EXERCISE

1. Write the key words in your notebook or on note cards. Write the words on one side of the notepaper and then write the definitions on the opposite side of the page or on the back of the paper. If using note cards, write the key word on the front and the definition on the back. *This step should be completed before the lab session begins.*

   Memorize the key word definitions silently for 5 minutes, then work with a lab partner and identify the words you still need help with. List the words here. Add additional rows if needed.

II. COMPREHENSION EXERCISE

1. Work with a lab partner to complete this exercise. For each laboratory value presented in the text, work with your partner to memorize the normal range for adults, two implications for low values, and two implications for high values.

   Alanine aminotransferase (ALT)
   Alpha fetoprotein
   Aspartate aminotransferase (AST)
   Amylase
   Bilirubin
   Blood urea nitrogen
   Cholesterol
   Creatine
   Creatine phosphokinase
   Estrogen
   Glucose
   Hematocrit
   Human chorionic gonadotropin (hCG)
   Lactate dehydrogenase (LD)
   Lipase
   Prostate-specific antigen (PSA)
   Thyroid-stimulating hormone (TSH)

III. APPLICATION OF ANATOMY AND PHYSIOLOGY EXERCISE

1. Using the table below, describe the location of each organ. What body system is it a part of? Use Chapter 5 if additional help is needed. What did you miss?

Review Table

Organ	Laboratory Test
Abdominal aorta	Hematocrit
Neonatal brain	
Liver	Bilirubin
Liver	ALT
Pancreas	AST
	ALP
	Total protein levels
Liver	LDL
Heart	HDL
	VLDL
	Total proteins
Liver	BUN
Kidney	Creatinine
Pancreas	Amylase
	Lipase
	Glucose
Heart	LD
	CPK
Male pelvis	PSA
Female pelvis	Estrogen (E1, E2, E3)
Obstetrics	hCG
	AFP
Thyroid gland	THS
Parathyroid gland	T3
	T4

2. Write two or three summary sentences for each system listed in question 1. Ask your lab partner to check your work. Now check your work against the explanations in the textbook. What else can you add to your description?

59

IV. CHAPTER EVALUATION EXERCISE

Based on your work with the chapter and its accompanying laboratory assignments, identify three concepts you believe are the most important. You may draw from any of the assignments you've already completed in the previous pages. Include a detailed rationale in your answers.

1. _____

   _____

   _____

2. _____

   _____

   _____

3. _____

   _____

   _____

Answer the questions below. Refer to page 370 for the answers.

Completion

1. High levels of _____ and _____ may be indicators the patient is alcoholic and may be the cause of liver damage.

2. The _____ is a non-governmental, voluntary agency that serves to ensure products, services, and systems have international safety, quality, and efficiency.

3. Human chorionic gonadotropin can be determined by blood or urine tests as early as _____ days post conception.

4. A patient should fast _____ hours prior to venipuncture to evaluate the lipase level.

5. _____ is commonly measured to monitor clotting levels when patents are taking blood-thinning medication.

6. hCG levels should _____ every 48 hours of early pregnancy.

7. AFP is produced in the fetal _____ and _____ of a developing fetus.

8. When cells of the body are damaged or destroyed, they release _____ into the blood.

9. Blood samples to evaluate lactic dehydrogenase in the cerebrospinal fluid are taken in the procedure called a _____.

10. _____ is a soft waxy substance found in all body parts and is needed for proper bodily function.

11. Creatine phosphokinase is an enzyme found in _____ tissues.

12. PSA levels are evaluated by obtaining _____ samples.

The Abdominal Aorta

I. MEMORIZATION EXERCISE

1. Write the key words in your notebook or on note cards. Write the words on one side of the notepaper and then write the definitions on the opposite side of the page or on the back of the paper. If using note cards, write the key word on the front and the definition on the back. *This step should be completed before the lab session begins.*

   Memorize the key word definitions silently for 5 minutes, then work with a lab partner and identify the words you still need help with. List the words here. Add additional rows if needed.

2. Next, write a short answer to the question just created.

   Example: "The aorta is a retroperitoneal vessel located slightly to the left of the spine. It leaves the heart and courses to the common iliac arteries in the pelvis. Its diameter should be no more than 3 cm at its widest point."

   Highlight or circle any part of your answers about which you are unsure, and check the answers in your textbook. If you are still unsure of the answers, put a question mark next to the answer(s) for the review session of the lab.

II. COMPREHENSION EXERCISE

1. Work with a lab partner to complete this exercise. You will need to write in your notebook. First, change each objective into a question.

   Example: "Describe the normal location, course, and size of the aorta" becomes "What are the normal location, course, and size of the aorta?"

61

III. ANATOMY APPLICATION EXERCISE

1. Label the aorta and its branches.

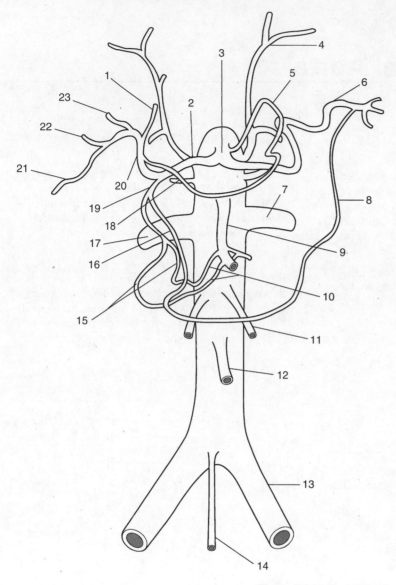

Figure 9-3 in the textbook

1	_____
2	_____
3	_____
4	_____
5	_____
6	_____
7	_____
8	_____
9	_____
10	_____
11	_____
12	_____
13	_____
14	_____
15	_____
16	_____
17	_____
18	_____
19	_____
20	_____
21	_____
22	_____
23	_____

2. Label the parts of the arterial wall.

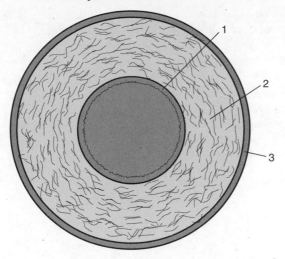

1 _____

2 _____

3 _____

Figure 9-4 in the textbook

3. Write two or three summary sentences on the physiology of the aorta. Check your work against the physiology section in the textbook. What else can you add to your description?

_____

_____

_____

IV. IMAGE ANALYSIS EXERCISE

Work on the following figures with your lab partner. It's your choice! You can label all the sketches at once, then go back and label each image with your lab partner, or label an image and its accompanying sketch at the same time. Either way, the goal is to label correctly all of the sketches and carefully compare the sketch with the sonographic image.

For each sonographic image, write a brief observation that could be "presented" to your instructor, a clinical sonographer, or a sonologist. Please review the section from Chapter 1 on How to Describe Ultrasound Findings. Remember that you want to:

- **differentiate** abnormal echo patterns from normal echo patterns,
- **document** any differences in echo pattern appearance, and
- **describe** any difference in echo pattern appearance using sonographic terminology.

For each image, your assessment should include (1) the view of each major structure (axial or longitudinal; note: these are not the scanning planes) and (2) structures identified in the image with correct sonographic appearance description and measurements if shown.

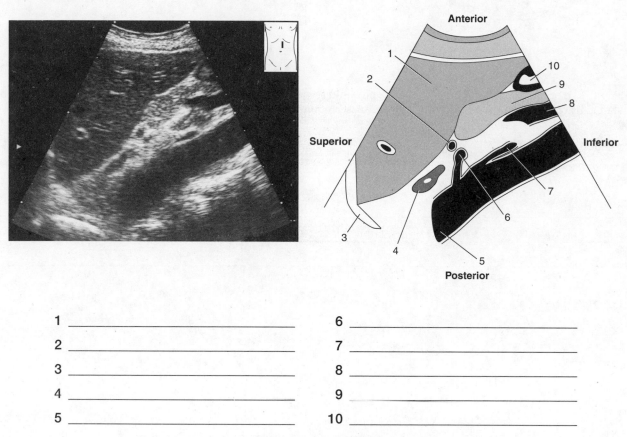

1 _____	6 _____
2 _____	7 _____
3 _____	8 _____
4 _____	9 _____
5 _____	10 _____

Figure 9-5 in the textbook

Description: _____

_____

_____

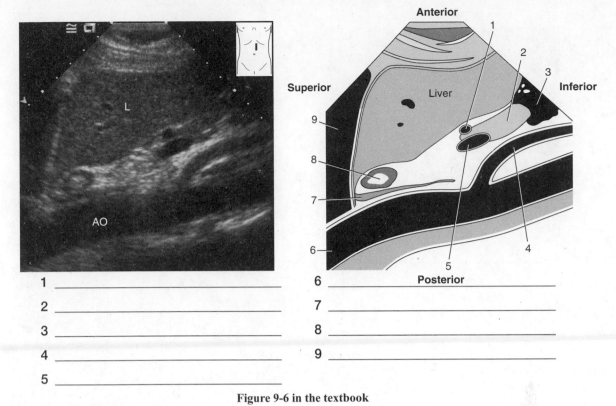

1	_____	6	_____
2	_____	7	_____
3	_____	8	_____
4	_____	9	_____
5	_____		

Figure 9-6 in the textbook

Description: _____

_____

_____

1	_____	5	_____
2	_____	6	_____
3	_____	7	_____
4	_____	8	_____

Figure 9-7 in the textbook

Description: _____

_____

_____

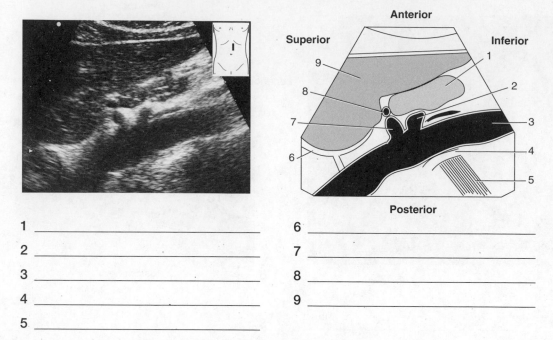

1 _____
2 _____
3 _____
4 _____
5 _____

6 _____
7 _____
8 _____
9 _____

Figure 9-8 in the textbook

Description: _____

_____

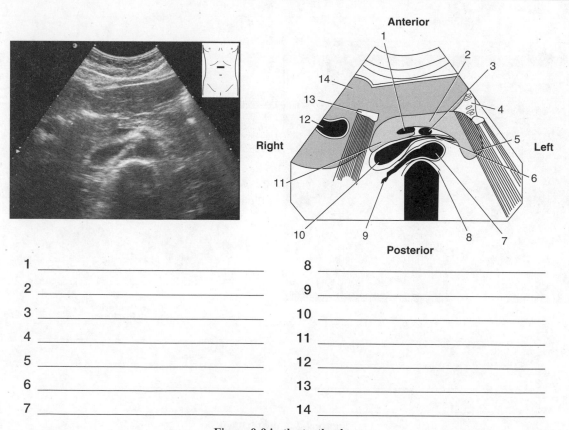

1 _____
2 _____
3 _____
4 _____
5 _____
6 _____
7 _____

8 _____
9 _____
10 _____
11 _____
12 _____
13 _____
14 _____

Figure 9-9 in the textbook

Description: _____

_____

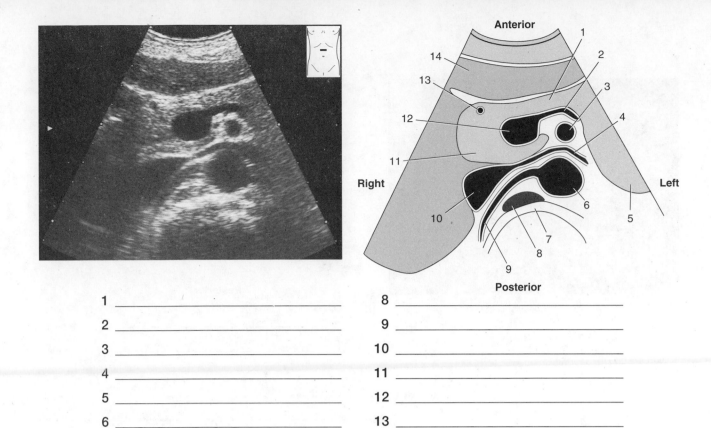

1	_____		8	_____
2	_____		9	_____
3	_____		10	_____
4	_____		11	_____
5	_____		12	_____
6	_____		13	_____
7	_____		14	_____

Figure 9-11 in the textbook

Description: _____

_____

_____

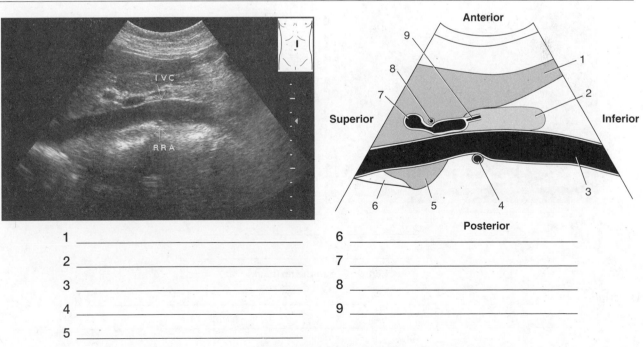

1	_____		6	_____
2	_____		7	_____
3	_____		8	_____
4	_____		9	_____
5	_____			

Figure 9-12 in the textbook

Description: _____

_____

_____

Chapter **9** **The Abdominal Aorta**

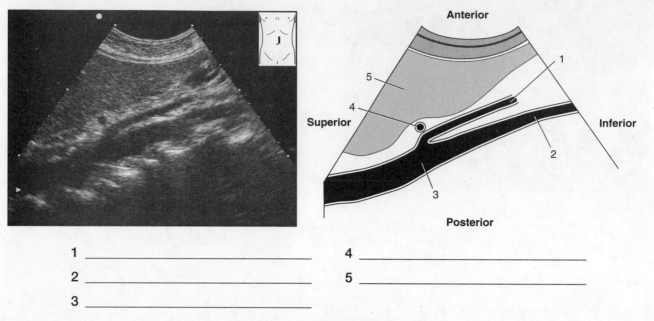

1 _____ 4 _____

2 _____ 5 _____

3 _____

Figure 9-13 in the textbook

Description: _____

_____

_____

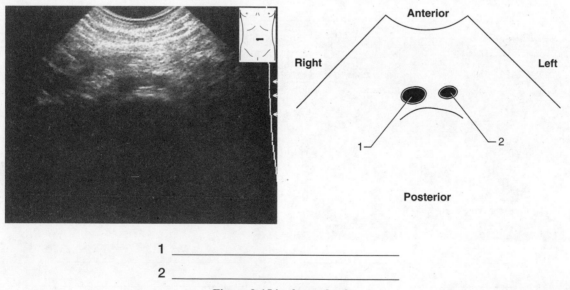

1 _____

2 _____

Figure 9-15 in the textbook

Description: _____

_____

_____

V. CHAPTER SUBHEADINGS EXERCISE

1. Convert each chapter subheading into a question; for example, change "Gross Anatomy" to "What is the gross anatomy of the aorta?" Write a brief answer to each question in a short paragraph in your notebook. Exchange answers with your lab partner and check each other's work. Refer back to the textbook for further information and explanation.

2. What questions about the chapter do you still have? Write your questions in your notebook.

VI. CHAPTER EVALUATION EXERCISE

Use a fresh sheet of notebook paper. Based on your work with the chapter and its accompanying laboratory assignments, identify three concepts you believe are the most important. You may draw from any of the assignments you've already completed in the previous pages, including learning objectives, anatomy and physiology, images, or chapter subheadings. Include a detailed rationale in your answers.

Answer the questions below. Refer to page 370 for the answers.

Multiple Choice

1. Which of the following vessels is seen sonographically as a linear structure that courses inferior and parallel to the aorta?
   a. Celiac artery
   b. Superior mesenteric artery
   c. Renal arteries
   d. Inferior mesenteric artery

2. Which of the following vessels are seen in a longitudinal course when the transducer is oriented in a transverse scanning plane?
   a. Hepatic arteries
   b. Gastric arteries
   c. Renal arteries
   d. Common iliac arteries

True/False

3. The celiac artery (CA) cannot be seen with reasonable consistency on ultrasound.

4. The anteroposterior measurement of the aorta should be obtained in an axial section to decrease variation among different sonographers.

5. The SMA demonstrates a high-resistance waveform in a patient who has not eaten.

6. The right gastric artery can originate from the proper hepatic artery, the gastroduodenal artery, or the common hepatic artery.

7. The right renal artery is longer than the left renal artery.

8. Longitudinal sections of the proximal portion of the abdominal aorta appear linear in configuration, and the mid and distal portions appear curvilinear.

9. The most inferior branch of the aorta is the inferior mesenteric artery.

10. Hematocrit measures how much of the total blood volume is red blood cells.

The Inferior Vena Cava

I. MEMORIZATION EXERCISE

1. Write the key words in your notebook or on note cards. Write the words on one side of the notepaper and then write the definitions on the opposite side of the page or on the back of the paper. If using note cards, write the key word on the front and the definition on the back. *This step should be completed before the lab session begins.*

   Memorize the key word definitions silently for 5 minutes, then work with a lab partner and identify the words you still need help with. List the words here. Add additional rows if needed.

II. COMPREHENSION EXERCISE

1. Work with a lab partner to complete this exercise. You will need to write in your notebook. First, change each objective into a question.

   Example: "Describe the normal location and course of the inferior vena cava" becomes "What are the normal location and course of the inferior vena cava?"

2. Next, write a short answer to the question just created.

   Example: "The inferior vena cava is a retroperitoneal vessel located slightly to the right of the spine. It begins at the union of the common iliac veins and empties into the right atrium of the heart."

   Highlight or circle any part of your answers about which you are unsure, and check the answers in your textbook. If you are still unsure of the answers, put a question mark next to the answer(s) for the review session of the lab.

III. ANATOMY APPLICATION EXERCISE

2. Write two or three summary sentences on the physiology of the inferior vena cava. Check your work against the physiology section of the textbook. What else can you add to your description?

_____

_____

_____

1. Label the IVC and its branches.

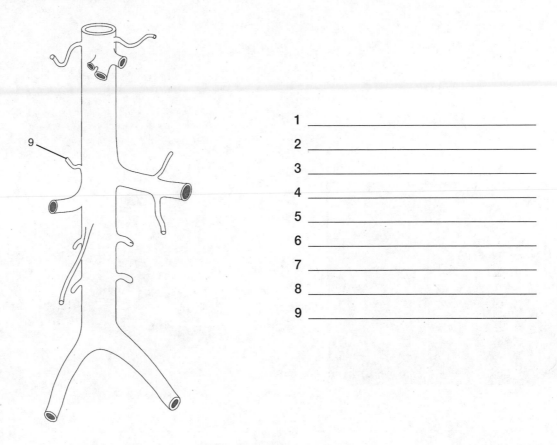

1 _____

2 _____

3 _____

4 _____

5 _____

6 _____

7 _____

8 _____

9 _____

Figure 10-2 in the textbook.

71

IV. IMAGE ANALYSIS EXERCISE

Work on the following figures with your lab partner. It's your choice! You can label all the sketches at once, then go back and label each image with your lab partner, or label an image and its accompanying sketch at the same time. Either way, the goal is to label correctly all of the sketches and carefully compare the sketch with the sonographic image.

For each sonographic image, write a brief observation that could be "presented" to your instructor, a clinical sonographer, or a sonologist. Please review the section from Chapter 1 on How to Describe Ultrasound Findings. Remember that you want to:

- **differentiate** abnormal echo patterns from normal echo patterns,
- **document** any differences in echo pattern appearance, and
- **describe** any difference in echo pattern appearance using sonographic terminology.

For each image, your assessment should include (1) the view of each major structure (axial or longitudinal; note: these are not the scanning planes) and (2) structures identified in the image with correct sonographic appearance description and measurements if shown.

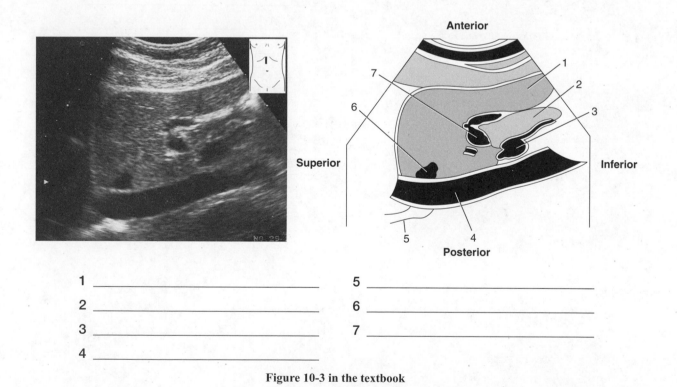

1 _____   5 _____

2 _____   6 _____

3 _____   7 _____

4 _____

Figure 10-3 in the textbook

Description: _____

_____

_____

Chapter **10**   **The Inferior Vena Cava**

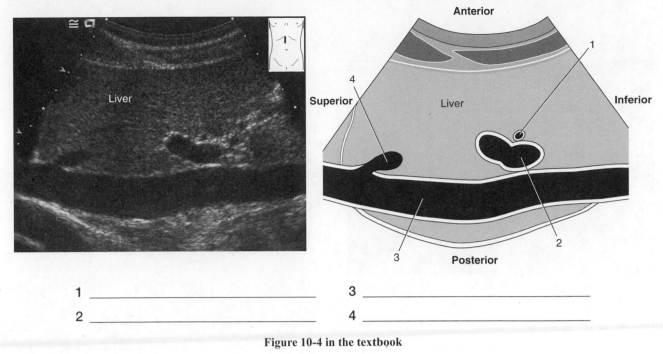

1	_____	3	_____
2	_____	4	_____

Figure 10-4 in the textbook

Description: _____

_____

_____

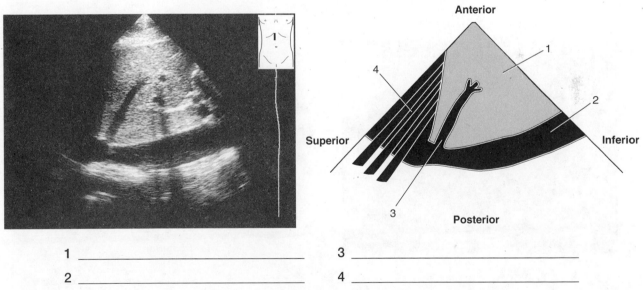

1	_____	3	_____
2	_____	4	_____

Figure 10-5 in the textbook

Description: _____

_____

_____

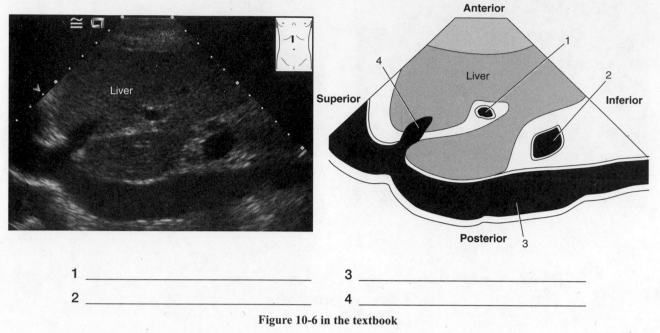

| 1 | _____ | 3 | _____ |
| 2 | _____ | 4 | _____ |

Figure 10-6 in the textbook

Description: _____

_____

_____

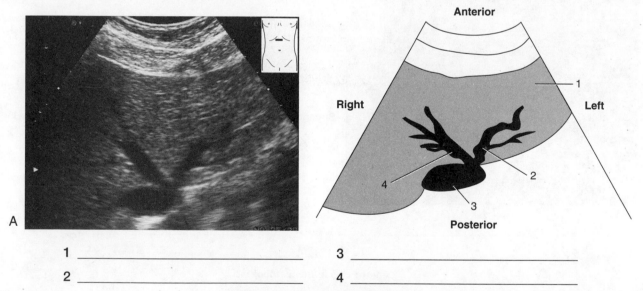

| 1 | _____ | 3 | _____ |
| 2 | _____ | 4 | _____ |

Figure 10-7A in the textbook

Description: _____

_____

_____

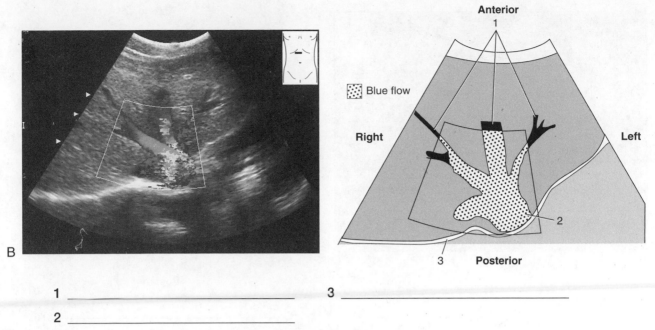

B

1 _____   3 _____

2 _____

Figure 10-7B in the textbook

Description: _____
_____
_____

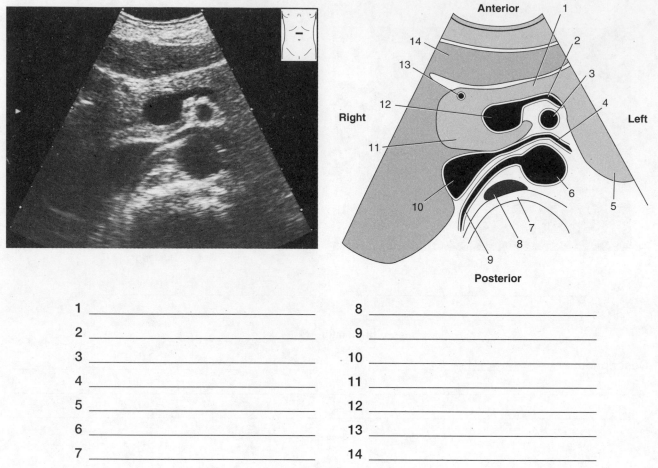

Figure 10-8 in the textbook

1 _____   8 _____

2 _____   9 _____

3 _____   10 _____

4 _____   11 _____

5 _____   12 _____

6 _____   13 _____

7 _____   14 _____

Description: _____

_____

_____

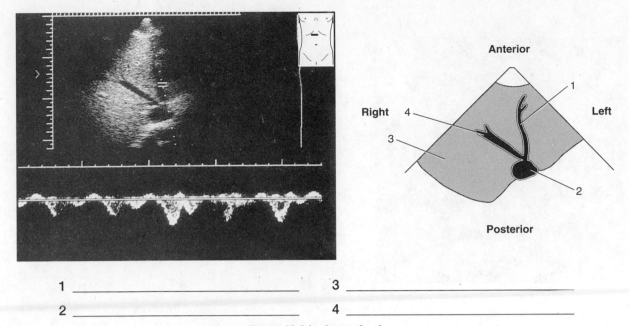

1 _____   3 _____

2 _____   4 _____

Figure 10-9 in the textbook

Description: _____
_____
_____

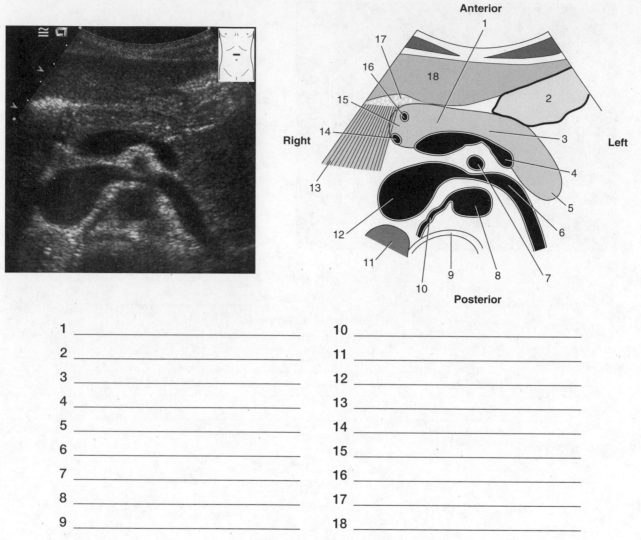

Figure 10-10 in the textbook

1	_____	10	_____
2	_____	11	_____
3	_____	12	_____
4	_____	13	_____
5	_____	14	_____
6	_____	15	_____
7	_____	16	_____
8	_____	17	_____
9	_____	18	_____

Description: _____

_____

_____

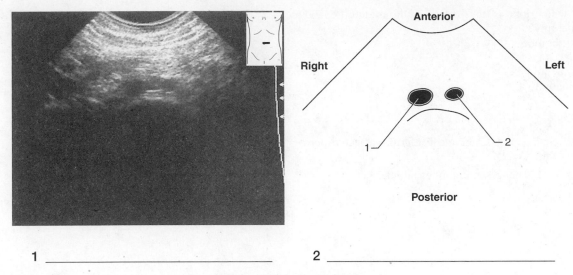

Figure 10-11 in the textbook

1 _____   2 _____

Description: _____

_____

_____

V. CHAPTER SUBHEADINGS EXERCISE

1. Convert each chapter subheading into a question; for example, change "Gross Anatomy" to "What is the gross anatomy of the inferior vena cava?" Write a brief answer to each question in a short paragraph in your notebook. Exchange answers with your lab partner and check each other's work. Refer back to the textbook for further information and explanation.
2. What questions do you still have about the chapter? Write your questions in your notebook.

VI. CHAPTER EVALUATION EXERCISE

Use a fresh sheet of notebook paper. Based on your work with the chapter and its accompanying laboratory assignments, identify three concepts you believe are the most important. You may draw from any of the assignments you've already completed in the previous pages, including learning objectives, anatomy and physiology, images, or chapter subheadings. Include a detailed rationale in your answers.

Answer the questions below. Refer to page 370 for the answers.

Multiple Choice

1. The IVC travels through the diaphragm and empties into the
   a. right atrium.
   b. left atrium.
   c. right ventricle.
   d. left ventricle.

2. Which portion of the IVC extends inferior to the hepatic veins and superior to the renal veins?
   a. Hepatic section
   b. Prerenal section
   c. Renal section
   d. Postrenal section

3. The left gonadal vein empties into the
   a. IVC.
   b. left renal vein.
   c. left suprarenal vein.
   d. left iliac vein.

4. Which is not a major tributary of the IVC?
   a. Hepatic veins
   b. Renal veins
   c. Portal veins
   d. Common iliac veins

5. Into which lobe of the liver does the middle hepatic vein empty?
   a. Right lobe
   b. Left lobe
   c. Caudate lobe
   d. Quadrate lobe

True/False

6. The renal section is the most inferiorly located portion of the IVC.

7. The right gonadal vein empties into the IVC.

8. The left common iliac vein is longer than the right common iliac vein.

9. The hepatic veins decrease in diameter as they approach the IVC.

10. Small, moving echoes visualized in the lumen of the IVC are a normal finding.

11 The Portal Venous System

I. MEMORIZATION EXERCISE

1. Write the key words in your notebook or on note cards. Write the words on one side of the notepaper and then write the definitions on the opposite side of the page or on the back of the paper. If using note cards, write the key word on the front and the definition on the back. *This step should be completed before the lab session begins.*

    Memorize the key word definitions silently for 5 minutes, then work with a lab partner and identify the words you still need help with. List the words here. Add additional rows if needed.

II. COMPREHENSION EXERCISE

1. Work with a lab partner to complete this exercise. You will need to write in your notebook. First, change each objective into a question.

    Example: "Describe the normal location, course, and size of the portal vein" becomes "What is the normal location, course, and size of the portal vein?"

2. Next, write a short answer to the question just created.

    Example: "The portal vein is an intraabdominal structure that drains the gastrointestinal tract. It courses from left to right and is formed near the head of the pancreas before entering the liver at the liver hilus. Its diameter is up to 13 mm, and its length is 5 to 6 cm."

    Highlight or circle any part of your answers about which you are unsure, and check the answers in your textbook. If you are still unsure of the answers, put a question mark next to the answer(s) for the review session of the lab.

III. APPLICATION OF ANATOMY AND PHYSIOLOGY EXERCISE

1. Label the portal vein and its branches

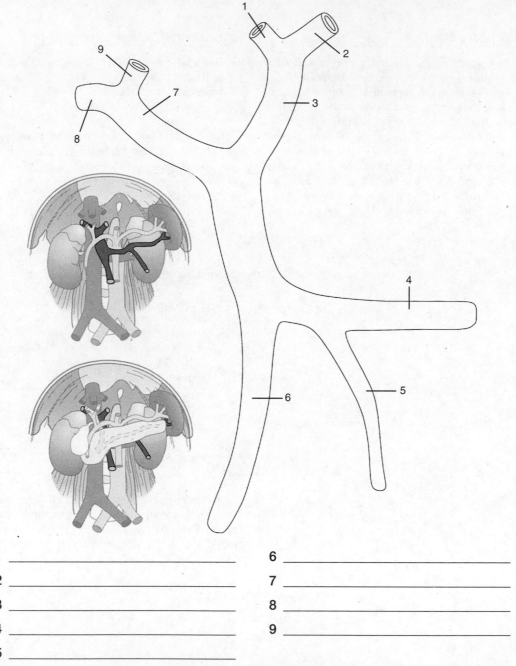

1 _____   6 _____

2 _____   7 _____

3 _____   8 _____

4 _____   9 _____

5 _____

Figure 11-1 in the textbook

2. Write two or three summary sentences of the physiology of the portal vein. Ask your lab partner to check your work. Now check your work against the physiology section in the textbook. What else can you add to your description?

_____

_____

_____

IV. IMAGE ANALYSIS EXERCISE

Work on the following figures with your lab partner. It's your choice! You can label all the sketches at once, then go back and label each image with your lab partner, or label an image and its accompanying sketch at the same time. Either way, the goal is to label correctly all of the sketches and carefully compare the sketch with the sonographic image.

For each sonographic image, write a brief observation that could be "presented" to your instructor, a clinical sonographer, or a sonologist. Please review the section from Chapter 1 on How to Describe Ultrasound Findings. Remember that you want to:

- **differentiate** abnormal echo patterns from normal echo patterns,
- **document** any differences in echo pattern appearance, and
- **describe** any difference in echo pattern appearance using sonographic terminology.

For each image, your assessment should include (1) the view of each major structure (axial or longitudinal; note: these are not the scanning planes) and (2) structures identified in the image with correct sonographic appearance description and measurements if shown.

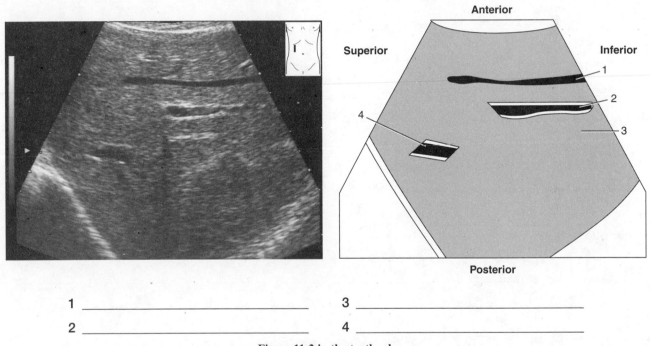

1 _____   3 _____

2 _____   4 _____

Figure 11-2 in the textbook

Description:

_____

_____

_____

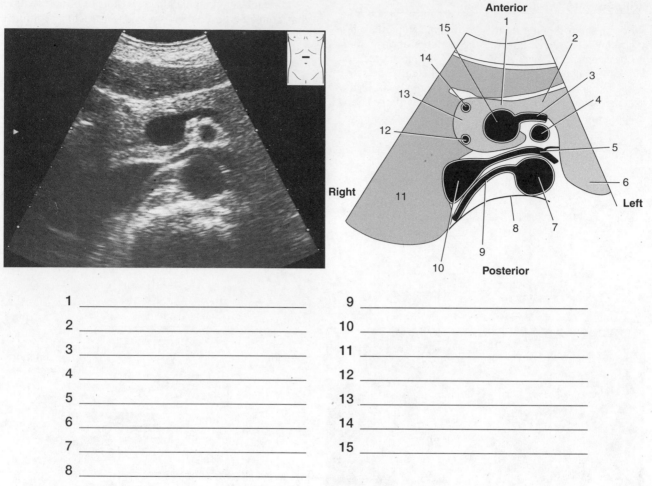

1	_____	9	_____
2	_____	10	_____
3	_____	11	_____
4	_____	12	_____
5	_____	13	_____
6	_____	14	_____
7	_____	15	_____
8	_____		

Figure 11-3 in the textbook

Description:

_____

_____

_____

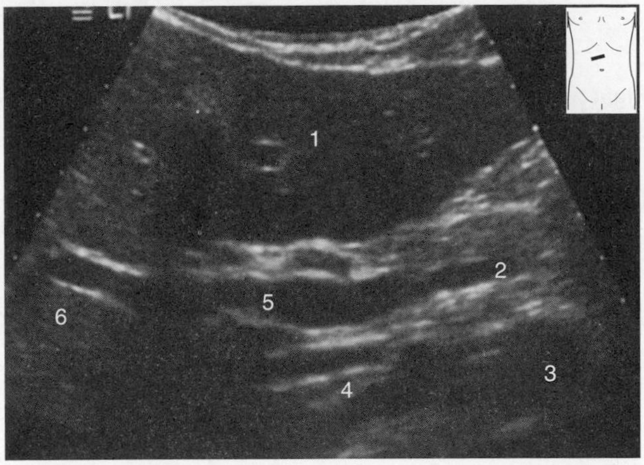

Figure 11-4 in the textbook

1 _____

2 _____

3 _____

4 _____

5 _____

6 _____

Description:

_____

_____

_____

A

1 _____   7 _____

2 _____   8 _____

3 _____   9 _____

4 _____   10 _____

5 _____   11 _____

6 _____

Figure 11-5A in the textbook

Description:

_____

_____

_____

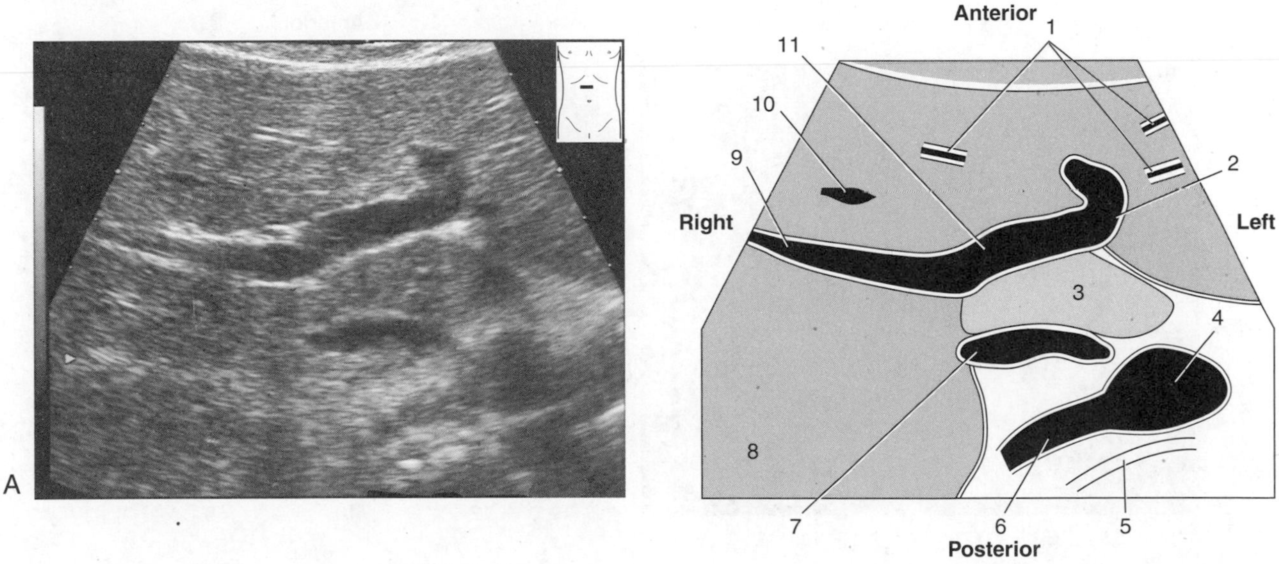

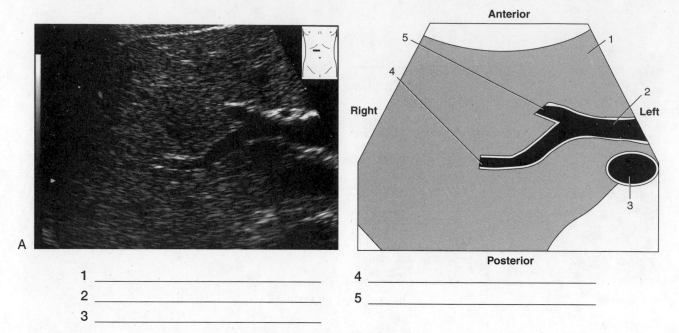

1 _____   4 _____
2 _____   5 _____
3 _____

Figure 11-7A in the textbook

Description:

_____

_____

_____

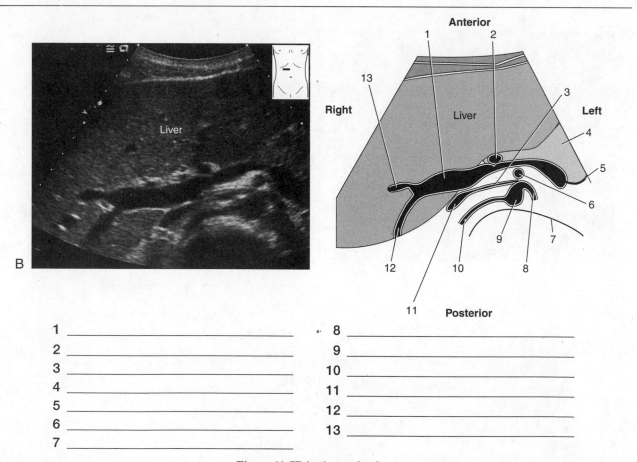

1 _____   8 _____
2 _____   9 _____
3 _____   10 _____
4 _____   11 _____
5 _____   12 _____
6 _____   13 _____
7 _____

Figure 11-7B in the textbook

Description:

_____

_____

_____

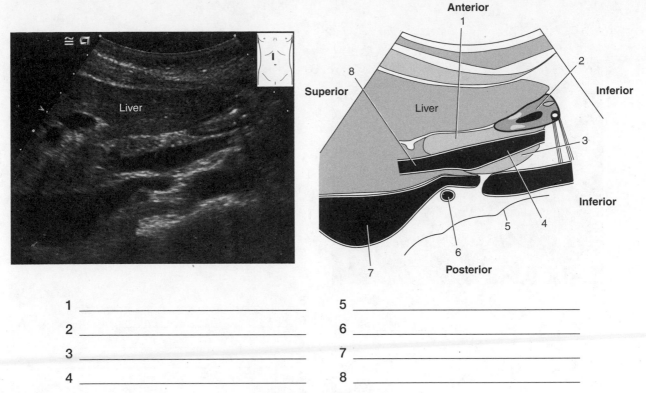

1 _____	5 _____
2 _____	6 _____
3 _____	7 _____
4 _____	8 _____

Figure 11-8 in the textbook

Description:

_____

_____

_____

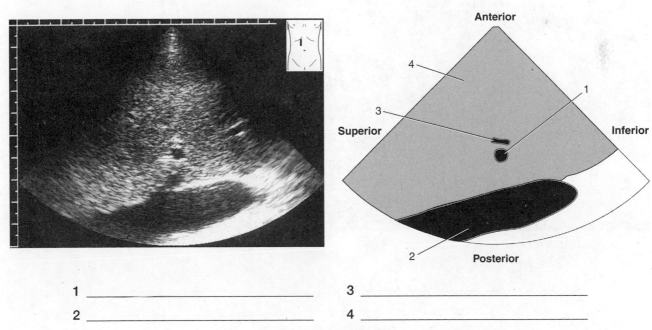

1 _____	3 _____
2 _____	4 _____

Figure 11-9 in the textbook

Description:

_____

_____

_____

Chapter **11** **The Portal Venous System**

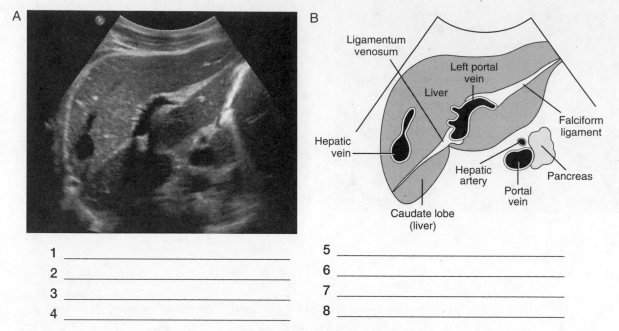

A

B

Ligamentum
venosum

Left portal
vein

Liver

Hepatic
vein

Falciform
ligament

Hepatic
artery

Portal
vein

Pancreas

Caudate lobe
(liver)

1 _____
2 _____
3 _____
4 _____

5 _____
6 _____
7 _____
8 _____

Figure 11-10 in the textbook

Description:

_____
_____
_____

Anterior

5

1

2

Superior

Inferior

4

3

Posterior

1 _____
2 _____
3 _____

4 _____
5 _____

Figure 11-11 in the textbook

Description:

_____
_____
_____

Chapter **11**   **The Portal Venous System**

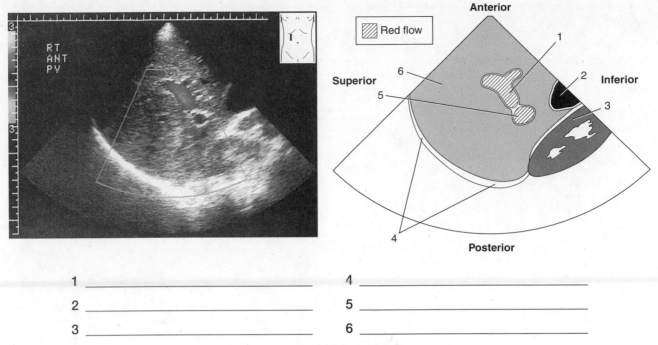

1 _____	4 _____
2 _____	5 _____
3 _____	6 _____

Figure 11-12 in the textbook

Description:

_____

_____

_____

V. CHAPTER SUBHEADINGS EXERCISE

1. Convert each chapter subheading into a question; for example, change "Gross Anatomy" to "What is the gross anatomy of the portal venous system?" Briefly write the answer to each question in a short paragraph in your notebook. Exchange answers with your lab partner and check each other's work. Refer back to the textbook for further information and explanation.

2. What questions do you still have about the chapter? Write your questions in your notebook.

VI. CHAPTER EVALUATION EXERCISE

Use a fresh sheet of notebook paper. Based on your work with the chapter and its accompanying laboratory assignments, identify three concepts you believe are the most important. You may draw from any of the assignments you have already completed in the previous pages including learning objectives, anatomy and physiology, images, or chapter subheadings. Include a detailed rationale in your answers.

Answer the questions below. Refer to page 370 for the answers.

True/False

1. The portal vein's walls appear distinctively brighter due to their high fat content and sheath covering.

2. The bifurcation of the right portal vein is best seen in the transverse scanning plane.

3. The union of the superior mesenteric vein and splenic vein is best appreciated in a sagittal scanning plane.

4. The portal vein courses 6 to 8 cm before bifurcating into right and left branches.

Completion

Indicate the primary path of the vessel as S (superior), IS (inferior to superior), LM (lateral to medial), R (to the right), or L (to the left).

5. Superior mesenteric vein _____.

6. Inferior mesenteric vein _____

7. Splenic vein _____

8. Right portal vein _____

9. Left portal vein _____

10. Portal vein _____

12 The Liver

I. MEMORIZATION EXERCISE

1. Write the key words in your notebook or on note cards. Write the words on one side of the notepaper and then write the definitions on the opposite side of the page or on the back of the paper. If using note cards, write the key word on the front and the definition on the back. *This step should be completed before the lab session begins.*

   Memorize the key word definitions silently for 5 minutes, then work with a lab partner and identify the words you still need help with. List the words here. Add additional rows if needed.

II. COMPREHENSION EXERCISE

1. Work with a lab partner to complete this exercise. You will need to write in your notebook. First, change each objective into a question.

   Example: "Describe the location of the liver" becomes "What is the location of the liver?"

2. Next, write a short answer to the question just created.

   Example: "The liver lies in the right hypochondrium. It extends inferiorly to the epigastrium and laterally to the left hypochondrium. Its superior portion reaches the diaphragm."

Highlight or circle any part of your answers about which you are unsure, and check the answers in your textbook. If you are still unsure of the answers, put a question mark next to the answer(s) for the review session of the lab.

III. APPLICATION OF ANATOMY AND PHYSIOLOGY EXERCISE

1. Label liver lobes.

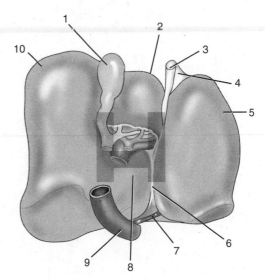

1 _____
2 _____
3 _____
4 _____
5 _____
6 _____
7 _____
8 _____
9 _____
10 _____

Figure 12-8, top, in the textbook

2. Label liver vasculature and surrounding anatomy and structures.

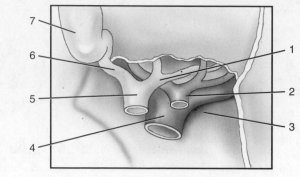

1 _____   5 _____

2 _____   6 _____

3 _____   7 _____

4 _____

Figure 12-8, bottom, in the textbook

3. Write two or three summary sentences of the physiology of the liver. Now check your work against the physiology section in the textbook. What else can you add to your description?

_____

_____

_____

IV. IMAGE ANALYSIS EXERCISE

Work on the following figures with your lab partner. It's your choice! You can label all the sketches at once, then go back and label each image with your lab partner, or label an image and its accompanying sketch at the same time. Either way, the goal is to label correctly all of the sketches and carefully compare the sketch with the sonographic image.

For each sonographic image, write a brief observation that could be "presented" to your instructor, a clinical sonographer, or a sonologist. Please review the section from Chapter 1 on How to Describe Ultrasound Findings. Remember that you want to:

- **differentiate** abnormal echo patterns from normal echo patterns,
- **document** any differences in echo pattern appearance, and
- **describe** any difference in echo pattern appearance using sonographic terminology.

For each image, your assessment should include (1) the view of each major structure (axial or longitudinal; note: these are not the scanning planes) and (2) structures identified in the image with correct sonographic appearance description and measurements if shown.

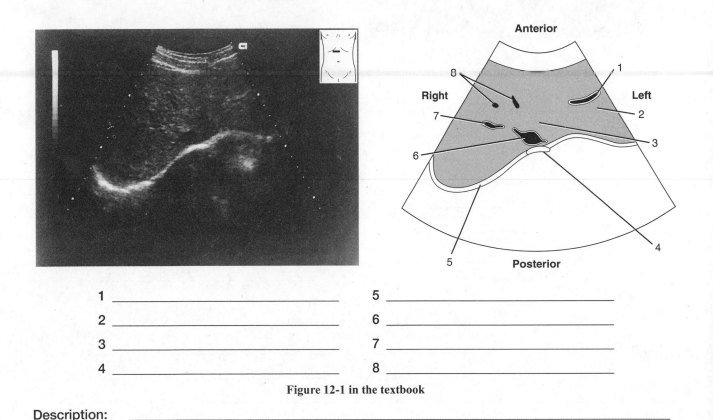

1 _____	5 _____
2 _____	6 _____
3 _____	7 _____
4 _____	8 _____

Figure 12-1 in the textbook

Description: _____

_____

_____

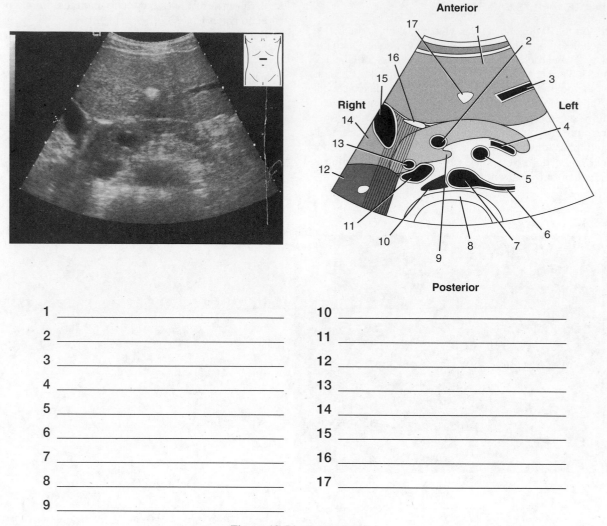

Figure 12-5 in the textbook

1 _____

2 _____

3 _____

4 _____

5 _____

6 _____

7 _____

8 _____

9 _____

10 _____

11 _____

12 _____

13 _____

14 _____

15 _____

16 _____

17 _____

Description: _____

_____

_____

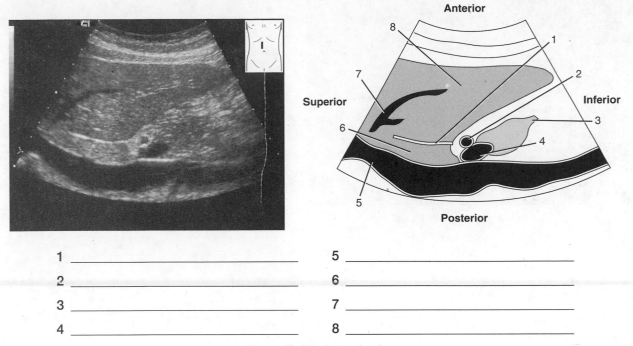

1	_____	5	_____
2	_____	6	_____
3	_____	7	_____
4	_____	8	_____

Figure 12-6 in the textbook

Description: _____

_____

_____

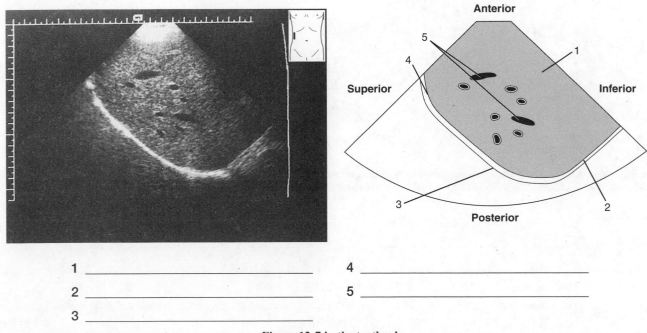

1	_____	4	_____
2	_____	5	_____
3	_____		

Figure 12-7 in the textbook

Description: _____

_____

_____

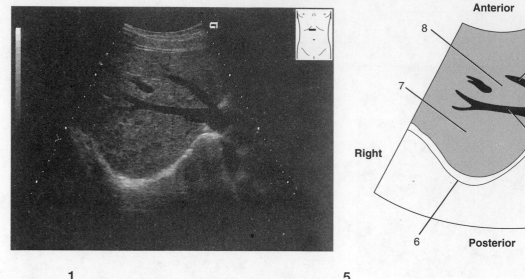

1	_____	5	_____
2	_____	6	_____
3	_____	7	_____
4	_____	8	_____

Figure 12-9 in the textbook

Description: _____

_____

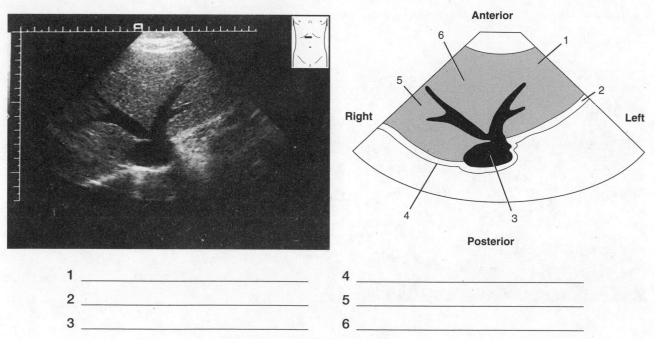

1	_____	4	_____
2	_____	5	_____
3	_____	6	_____

Figure 12-10 in the textbook

Description: _____

_____

Chapter **12** **The Liver**

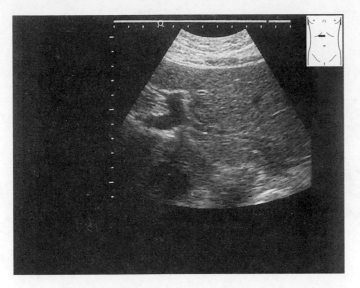
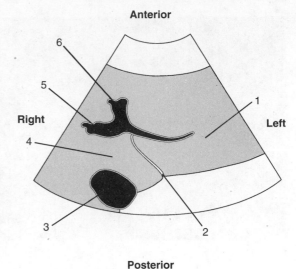

1	_____	4	_____
2	_____	5	_____
3	_____	6	_____

Figure 12-11 in the textbook

Description: _____

_____

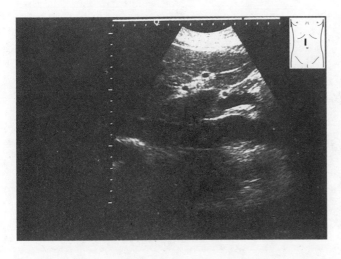
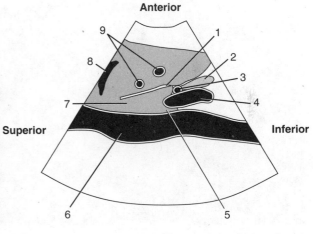

1	_____	6	_____
2	_____	7	_____
3	_____	8	_____
4	_____	9	_____
5	_____		

Figure 12-12 in the textbook

Description: _____

_____

_____

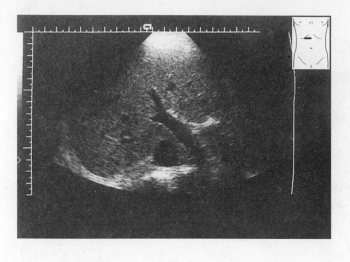
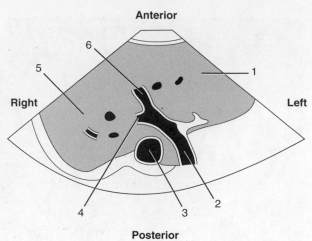

1	_____	4	_____
2	_____	5	_____
3	_____	6	_____

Figure 12-13 in the textbook

Description: _____

_____

_____

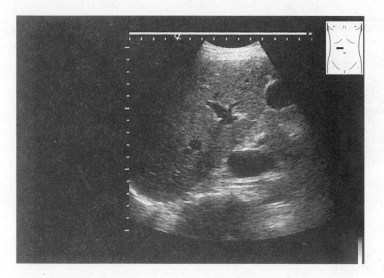
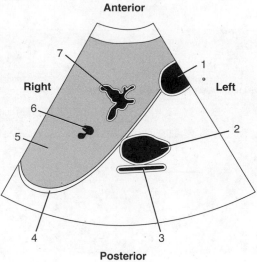

1	_____	5	_____
2	_____	6	_____
3	_____	7	_____
4	_____		

Figure 12-14 in the textbook

Description: _____

_____

_____

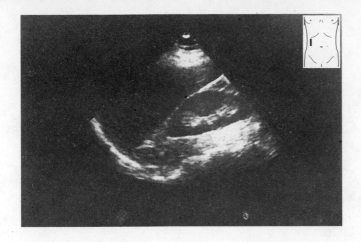
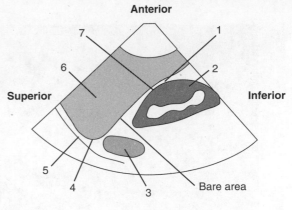

1	_____	5	_____
2	_____	6	_____
3	_____	7	_____
4	_____		

Figure 12-15 in the textbook

Description: _____

_____

_____

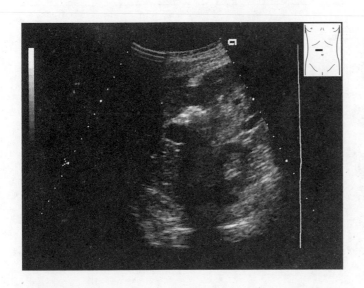
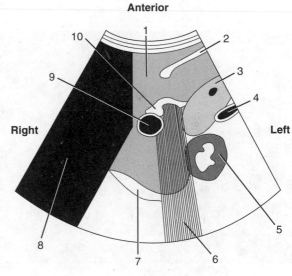

1	_____	6	_____
2	_____	7	_____
3	_____	8	_____
4	_____	9	_____
5	_____	10	_____

Figure 12-16 in the textbook

Description: _____

_____

_____

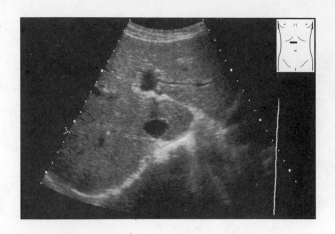

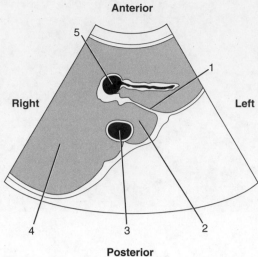

Anterior

5

1

Right

Left

4

3

2

Posterior

1 _____   4 _____

2 _____   5 _____

3 _____

Figure 12-17 in the textbook

Description: _____

_____

_____

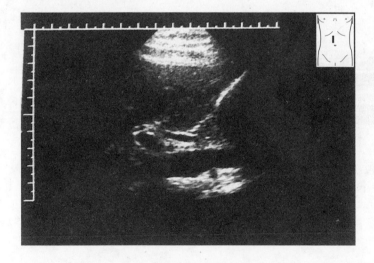

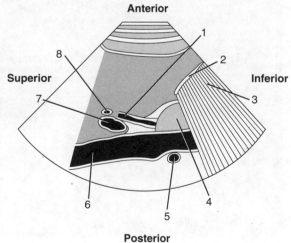

Anterior

8

1

2

Superior

Inferior

7

3

6

5

4

Posterior

1 _____   5 _____

2 _____   6 _____

3 _____   7 _____

4 _____   8 _____

Figure 12-18 in the textbook

Description: _____

_____

_____

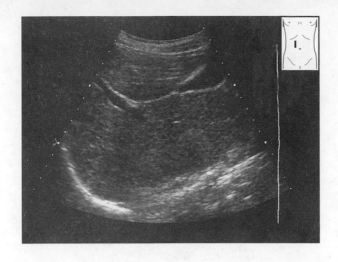
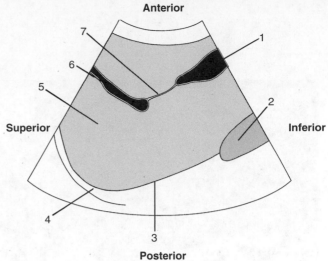

1	_____	5	_____
2	_____	6	_____
3	_____	7	_____
4	_____		

Figure 12-19 in the textbook

Description: _____

_____

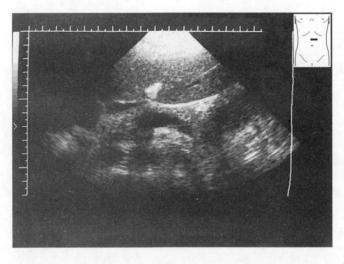
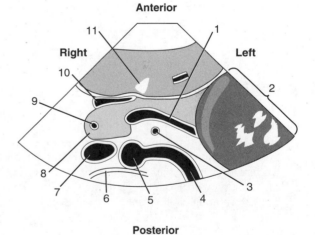

1	_____	7	_____
2	_____	8	_____
3	_____	9	_____
4	_____	10	_____
5	_____	11	_____
6	_____		

Figure 12-20 in the textbook

Description: _____

_____

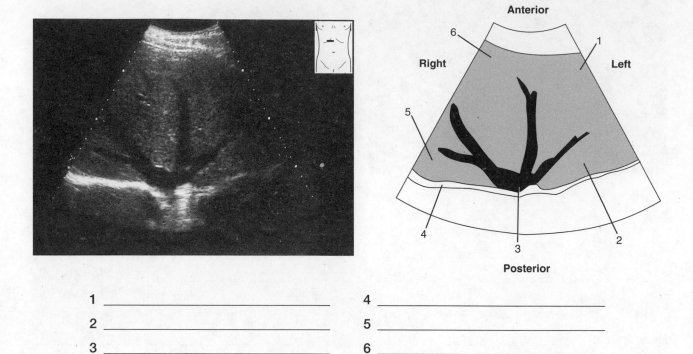

Anterior

Right   Left

6   1

5

4   3   2

Posterior

1	_____	4	_____
2	_____	5	_____
3	_____	6	_____

Figure 12-21 in the textbook

Description: _____

_____

_____

V. CHAPTER SUBHEADINGS EXERCISE

1. Convert each chapter subheading into a question; for example, change "Gross Anatomy" to "What is the gross anatomy of the liver?" Briefly write the answer to each question in a short paragraph in your notebook. Exchange answers with your lab partner and check each other's work. Refer back to the textbook for further information and explanation.

2. What questions do you still have about the chapter? Write your questions in your notebook.

VI. CHAPTER EVALUATION EXERCISE

Use a fresh sheet of notebook paper. Based on your work with the chapter and its accompanying laboratory assignments, identify three concepts you believe are the most important. You may draw from any of the assignments you have already completed in the previous pages including learning objectives, anatomy and physiology, images, or chapter subheadings. Include a detailed rationale in your answers.

Answer the questions below. Refer to page 370 for the answers.

Multiple Choice

1. The section of liver that is not covered by peritoneum is called the
   a. caudate lobe.
   b. bare area.
   c. mid clavicular line.
   d. medial left lobe.

2. The omental bursa is identified by its location posterior to the stomach and anterior to the pancreas and transverse colon. Another name for this bursa is the
   a. falciform ligament.
   b. greater sac.
   c. lesser sac.
   d. Morrison's pouch.

3. The area of the liver hilum where the portal vein enters and the common bile duct exits is called the
   a. porta hepatis.
   b. portal confluence.
   c. subhepatic space.
   d. subphrenic space.

4. Liver structures such as the hepatic ligaments and fissures, arteries, portal and hepatic veins and ducts are easily identifiable structures that help divide the liver into segments.
   a. True
   b. False

5. Which of the following liver surfaces would not be in contact with the diaphragm?
   a. The superior surface
   b. The inferior surface
   c. The anterior surface
   d. The bare area

6. The surface of the liver marked with indentations and in contact with abdominal organs is the
   a. superior surface.
   b. inferior surface.
   c. anterior surface.
   d. bare area.

7. Which of the following ligaments or fissures marks the left lateral boundary of the medial portion of the left liver lobe?
   a. Hepatoduodenal ligament
   b. Coronary ligament
   c. Falciform ligament
   d. Main lobar fissure

8. A large left lobe of the liver would be helpful in visualizing which of the following structures?
   a. Pancreas
   b. Ascending colon
   c. Veriform appendix
   d. Right portal vein

9. The right and left lobes of the liver are divided into four segments, medial and lateral on the right and anterior and posterior on the left.
   a. True
   b. False

10. Which of the following is another term for the medial segment of the left lobe?
    a. Caudate lobe
    b. Quadrate lobe
    c. Reidel's lobe
    d. Posterior portion of the inferior surface

The Biliary System 13

I. MEMORIZATION EXERCISE

1. Write the key words in your notebook or on note cards. Write the words on one side of the notepaper and then write the definitions on the opposite side of the page or on the back of the paper. If using note cards, write the key word on the front and the definition on the back. *This step should be completed before the lab session begins.*

   Memorize the key word definitions silently for 5 minutes, then work with a lab partner and identify the words you still need help with. List the words here. Add additional rows if needed.

II. COMPREHENSION EXERCISE

1. Work with a lab partner to complete this exercise. You will need to write in your notebook. First, change each objective into a question.

   Example: "Describe the basic function of the biliary system" becomes "What is the basic function of the biliary system?"

2. Next, write a short answer to the question just created.

   Example: "The biliary system conveys bile, manufactured in the liver, from the liver to the gallbladder for storage. The hormone cholecystokinin stimulates release of the bile from the gallbladder to the duodenum. Bile is transported to the duodenum via the common bile duct and enters the duodenum through the sphincter of Oddi. The purpose of bile is to help break down fats in the duodenum, aiding digestion."

   Highlight or circle any part of your answers about which you are unsure, and check the answers in your textbook. If you are still unsure of the answers, put a question mark next to the answer(s) for the review session of the lab.

III. APPLICATION OF ANATOMY AND PHYSIOLOGY EXERCISE

1. Label the biliary system.

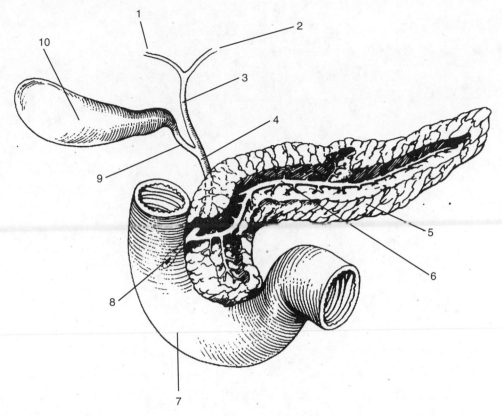

Figure 13-2 in the textbook

1 _____   6 _____

2 _____   7 _____

3 _____   8 _____

4 _____   9 _____

5 _____   10 _____

2. Label the gallbladder and surrounding vasculature.

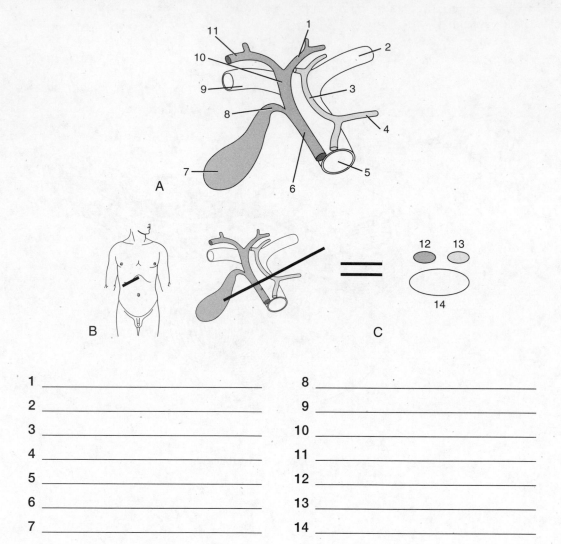

A

B

C

1 _____
2 _____
3 _____
4 _____
5 _____
6 _____
7 _____

8 _____
9 _____
10 _____
11 _____
12 _____
13 _____
14 _____

3. Write two or three summary sentences of the physiology of the biliary system. Now check your work against the physiology section in the textbook. What else can you add to your description?

_____

_____

_____

IV. IMAGE ANALYSIS EXERCISE

Work on the following figures with your lab partner. It's your choice! You can label all the sketches at once, then go back and label each image with your lab partner, or label an image and its accompanying sketch at the same time. Either way, the goal is to label correctly all of the sketches and carefully compare the sketch with the sonographic image.

For each sonographic image, write a brief observation that could be "presented" to your instructor, a clinical sonographer, or a sonologist. Please review the section from Chapter 1 on How to Describe Ultrasound Findings. Remember that you want to:

- **differentiate** abnormal echo patterns from normal echo patterns,
- **document** any differences in echo pattern appearance, and
- **describe** any difference in echo pattern appearance using sonographic terminology.

For each image, your assessment should include (1) the view of each major structure (axial or longitudinal; note: these are not the scanning planes) and (2) structures identified in the image with correct sonographic appearance description and measurements if shown.

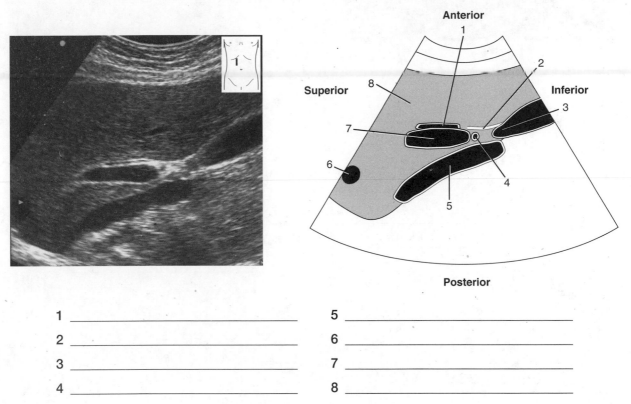

1	_____	5	_____
2	_____	6	_____
3	_____	7	_____
4	_____	8	_____

Figure 13-1 in the textbook

Description: _____

_____

_____

_____

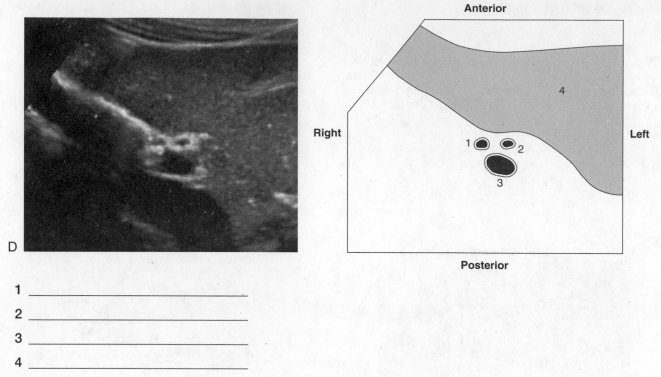

D

Anterior

Right

Left

Posterior

1 _____

2 _____

3 _____

4 _____

Figure 13-4D in the textbook

Description: _____
_____
_____
_____

Chapter **13** **The Biliary System**

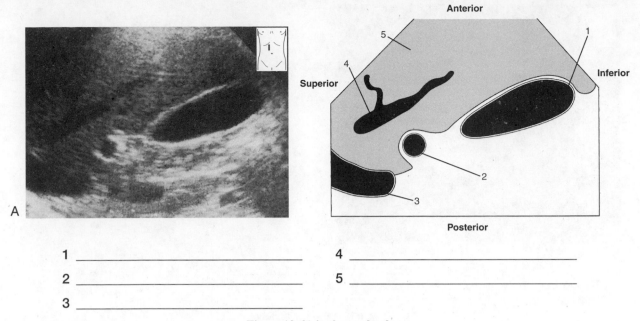

1	_____	4	_____
2	_____	5	_____
3	_____		

Figure 13-6A in the textbook

Description: _____

_____

_____

_____

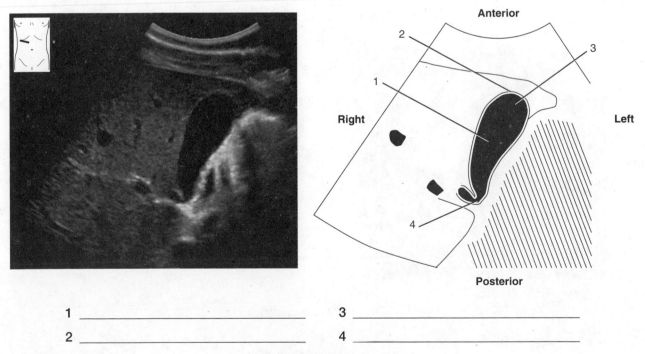

| 1 | _____ | 3 | _____ |
| 2 | _____ | 4 | _____ |

Figure 13-8 in the textbook

Description: _____

_____

_____

_____

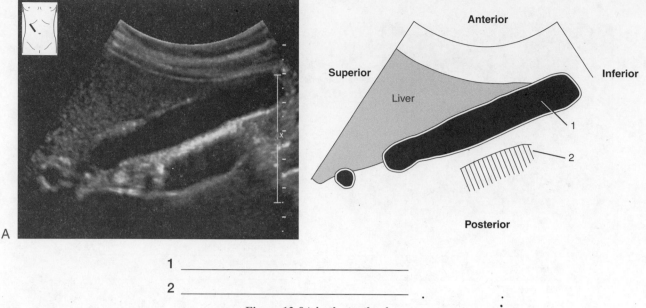

1 _____

2 _____   .   :

Figure 13-9A in the textbook

Description: _____

_____

_____

_____

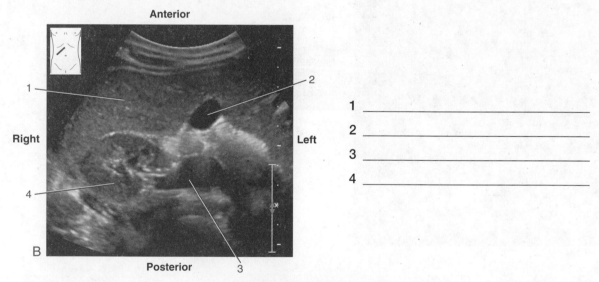

1 _____

2 _____

3 _____

4 _____

Figure 13-9B in the textbook

Description: _____

_____

_____

_____

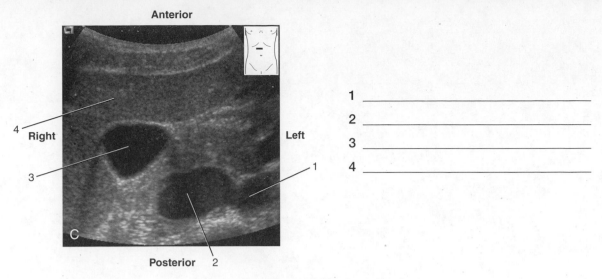

Anterior

Right   Left

Posterior

1 _____
2 _____
3 _____
4 _____

Figure 13-9C in the textbook

Description: _____

_____

_____

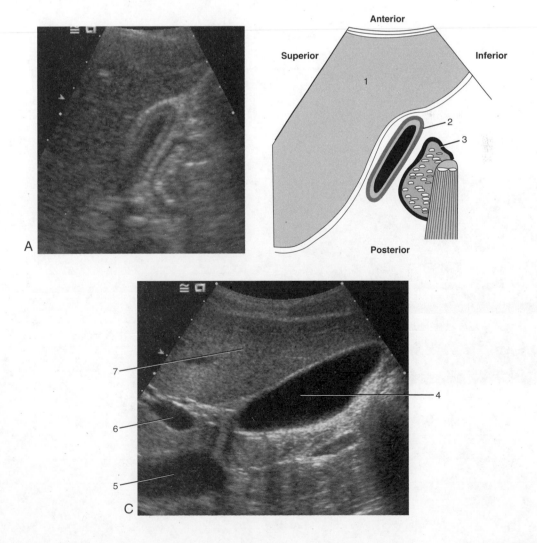

Anterior

Superior   Inferior

Posterior

1 _____   5 _____

2 _____   6 _____

3 _____   7 _____

4 _____

Figure 13-10A and C in the textbook

Description for A:

_____

_____

_____

Description for C:

_____

_____

_____

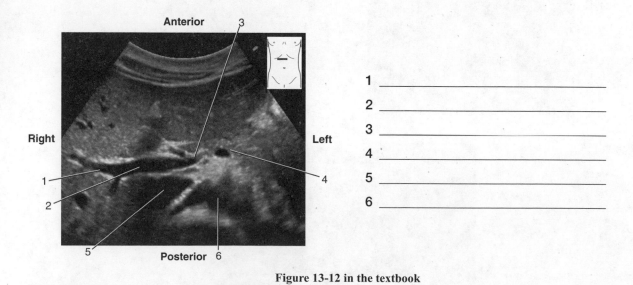

1 _____

2 _____

3 _____

4 _____

5 _____

6 _____

Figure 13-12 in the textbook

Description: _____

_____

_____

_____

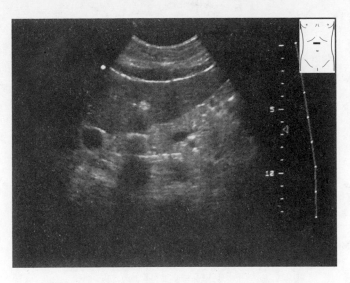 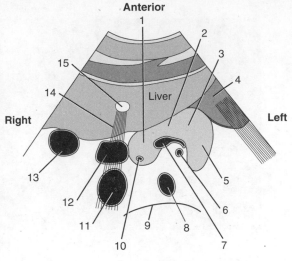

1	_____	9	_____
2	_____	10	_____
3	_____	11	_____
4	_____	12	_____
5	_____	13	_____
6	_____	14	_____
7	_____	15	_____
8	_____		

Figure 13-13 in the textbook

Description: _____

_____

_____

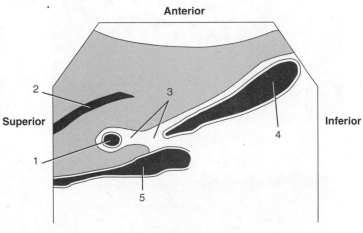

1	_____		
2	_____	4	_____
3	_____	5	_____

Figure 13-14 in the textbook

Description: _____

_____

_____

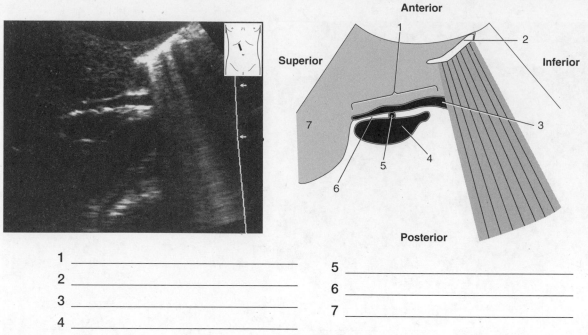

Anterior

Superior / Inferior

1, 2, 3, 4, 5, 6, 7

Posterior

1 _____	5 _____
2 _____	6 _____
3 _____	7 _____
4 _____	

Figure 13-18 in the textbook

Description: _____

_____

_____

_____

Anterior

Right / Left

1, 2, 3, 4, 5, 6, 7, 8, 9, 10, 11, 12, 13, 14, 15

Posterior

1 _____	9 _____
2 _____	10 _____
3 _____	11 _____
4 _____	12 _____
5 _____	13 _____
6 _____	14 _____
7 _____	15 _____
8 _____	

Figure 13-19 in the textbook

Description: _____

_____

_____

V. CHAPTER SUBHEADINGS EXERCISE

1. Convert each chapter subheading into a question; for example, change "Gross Anatomy" to "What is the gross anatomy of the biliary system?" Write the answer to each question in a short paragraph in your notebook. Exchange answers with your lab partner and check each other's work. Refer back to the textbook for further information and explanation.

2. What questions do you still have about the chapter? Write your questions in your notebook.

VI. CHAPTER EVALUATION EXERCISE

Use a fresh sheet of notebook paper. Based on your work with the chapter and its accompanying laboratory assignments, identify three concepts you believe are the most important. You may draw from any of the assignments you have already completed in the previous pages including learning objectives, anatomy and physiology, images, or chapter subheadings. Include a detailed rationale in your answers.

Answer the questions below. Refer to page 370 for the answers.

Multiple Choice

1. Which maximum measurement is noted for a bile-filled gallbladder?
   a. 12 cm
   b. 5 cm
   c. 9 cm
   d. 15 cm

2. Which aspect of the common duct is considered the common bile duct?
   a. Proximal
   b. Superior
   c. Distal
   d. Anterior

3. Which congenital sonographic finding can appear similar to an hourglass?
   a. Duplicated gallbladder
   b. Phrygian cap
   c. Junctional fold
   d. Bilobed

4. Which sonographic finding is associated with the presence of stones in the ductal system?
   a. Cholelithiasis
   b. Choledocholithiasis
   c. Nephrocalcinosis
   d. Sludge

5. Which clinical indication presents as yellowish skin?
   a. Jaundice
   b. Cyanosis
   c. Pallor
   d. Erythema

6. Which imaging test is used to assess the function of the gallbladder?
   a. HIDA scan
   b. CT scan
   c. OCG
   d. ERCP

7. Which term best characterizes the widest portion of the gallbladder?
   a. Neck
   b. Body
   c. Tail
   d. Fundus

8. Which group of terms is associated with an extrahepatic portal triad?
   a. Right portal vein, common bile duct, and cystic artery
   b. Main portal vein, proper hepatic artery, and common bile duct
   c. Left portal vein, left hepatic artery, and common bile duct
   d. Main portal vein, common hepatic duct, and main hepatic artery

9. Which sonographic feature best characterizes a choledochal cyst?
   a. Outpouching of the gallbladder neck
   b. Dilatation of the common bile duct
   c. Pedunculated areas around the gallbladder fundus
   d. Dilatation of the cystic duct

10. Which muscle sheath regulates the flow of bile into the duodenum?
    a. Ampulla of Vater
    b. Rectus abdominis muscle
    c. Sphincter of Oddi
    d. Pylorus

I. MEMORIZATION EXERCISE

1. Write the key words in your notebook or on note cards. Write the words on one side of the notepaper and then write the definitions on the opposite side of the page or on the back of the paper. If using note cards, write the key word on the front and the definition on the back. *This step should be completed before the lab session begins.*

   Memorize the key word definitions silently for 5 minutes, then work with a lab partner and identify the words you still need help with. List the words here. Add additional rows if needed.

II. COMPREHENSION EXERCISE

1. Work with a lab partner to complete this exercise. You will need to write in your notebook. First, change each objective into a question.

> *Example:* "Describe the basic function of the pancreas" becomes "What is the basic function of the pancreas?"

2. Next, write a short answer to the question just created.

> *Example:* "The pancreas is an endocrine and exocrine organ. Only 2% of the gland's weight is for its endocrine function. The endocrine function is to produce insulin, glucagon, and somatostatin to regulate blood glucose. The exocrine function is to produce pancreatic juice, a substance that helps digest fats, proteins, carbohydrates, and nucleic acids."

Highlight or circle any part of your answers about which you are unsure, and check the answers in your textbook. If you are still unsure of the answers, put a question mark next to the answer(s) for the review session of the lab.

III. APPLICATION OF ANATOMY AND PHYSIOLOGY EXERCISE

1. Label the pancreas and the surrounding vasculature.

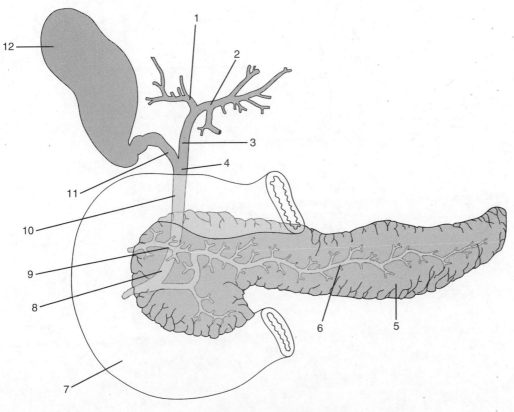

Figure 14-1 in the textbook

2. Write two or three summary sentences on the physiology of the pancreas. Now check your work against the physiology section of the textbook. What else can you add to your description?

_____

_____

_____

_____

_____

IV. IMAGE ANALYSIS EXERCISE

Work on the following figures with your lab partner. It's your choice! You can label all the sketches at once, then go back and label each image with your lab partner, or label an image and its accompanying sketch at the same time. Either way, the goal is to label correctly all of the sketches and carefully compare the sketch with the sonographic image.

For each sonographic image, write a brief observation that could be "presented" to your instructor, a clinical sonographer, or a sonologist. Please review the section from Chapter 1 on How to Describe Ultrasound Findings. Remember that you want to:

- **differentiate** abnormal echo patterns from normal echo patterns,
- **document** any differences in echo pattern appearance, and
- **describe** any difference in echo pattern appearance using sonographic terminology.

For each image, your assessment should include (1) the view of each major structure (axial or longitudinal; note: these are not the scanning planes) and (2) structures identified in the image with correct sonographic appearance description and measurements if shown.

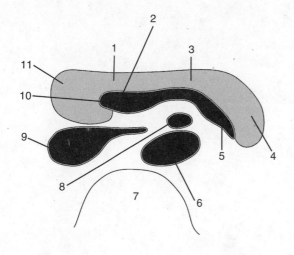

1 _____

2 _____

3 _____

4 _____

5 _____

6 _____

7 _____

8 _____

9 _____

10 _____

11 _____

Figure 14-2 in the textbook

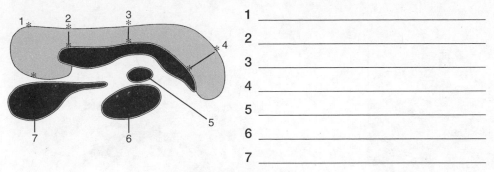

Figure 14-3 in the textbook

1	_____
2	_____
3	_____
4	_____
5	_____
6	_____
7	_____

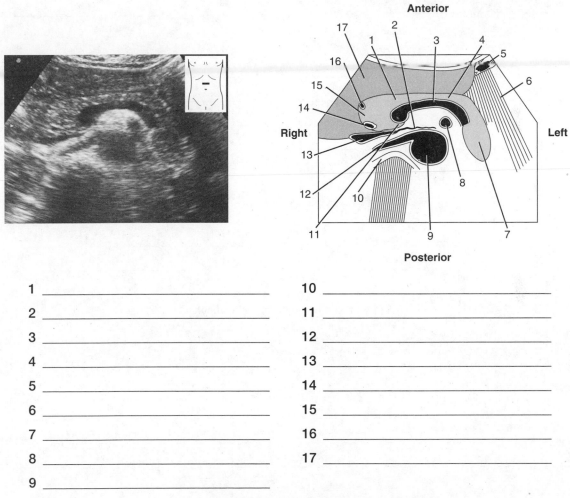

Figure 14-7, top, in the textbook

1	_____		10	_____
2	_____		11	_____
3	_____		12	_____
4	_____		13	_____
5	_____		14	_____
6	_____		15	_____
7	_____		16	_____
8	_____		17	_____
9	_____			

Description:

_____

_____

_____

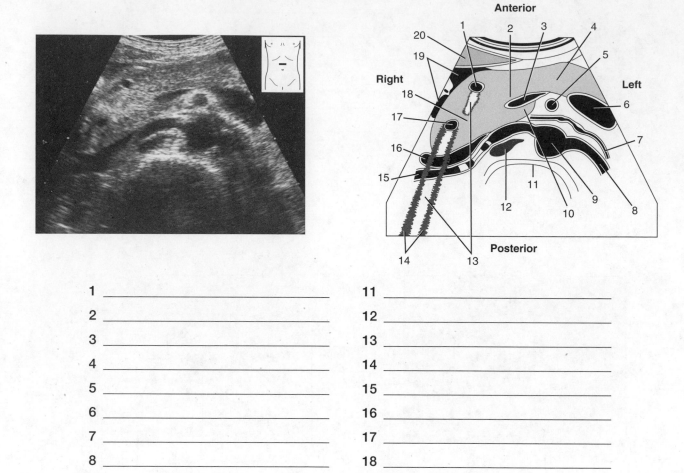

Figure 14-7, middle, in the textbook

1 _____	11 _____
2 _____	12 _____
3 _____	13 _____
4 _____	14 _____
5 _____	15 _____
6 _____	16 _____
7 _____	17 _____
8 _____	18 _____
9 _____	19 _____
10 _____	20 _____

Description:

_____

_____

_____

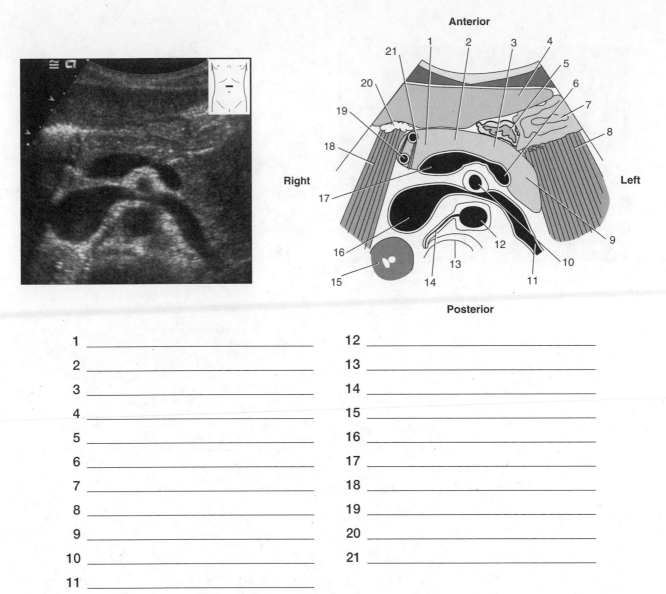

Figure 14-7, bottom, in the textbook

1	12	
2	13	
3	14	
4	15	
5	16	
6	17	
7	18	
8	19	
9	20	
10	21	
11		

Description:

_____

_____

_____

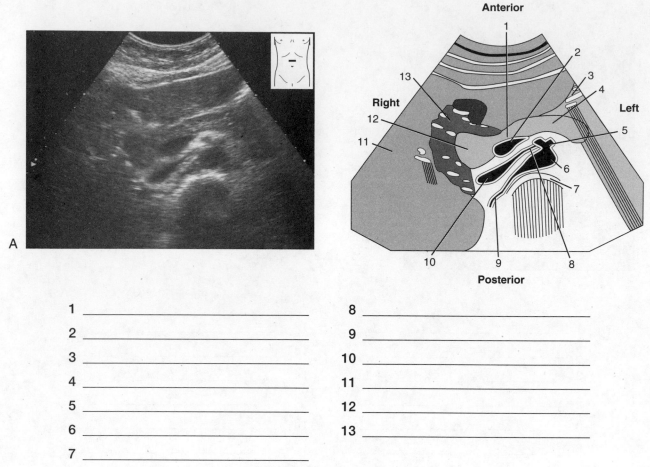

Figure 14-8A in the textbook

1	_____	8	_____
2	_____	9	_____
3	_____	10	_____
4	_____	11	_____
5	_____	12	_____
6	_____	13	_____
7	_____		

Description:

_____

_____

_____

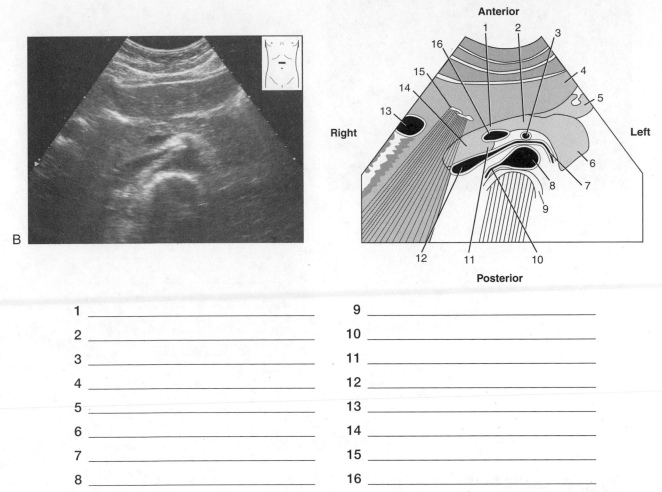

Figure 14-8B in the textbook

1 _____	9 _____
2 _____	10 _____
3 _____	11 _____
4 _____	12 _____
5 _____	13 _____
6 _____	14 _____
7 _____	15 _____
8 _____	16 _____

Description:

_____

_____

_____

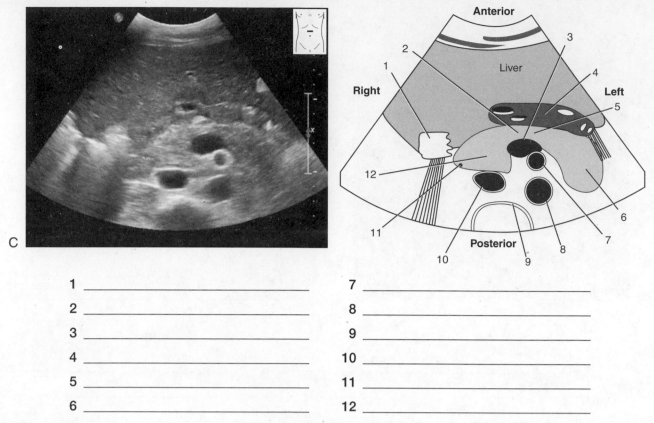

C

1	_____	7	_____
2	_____	8	_____
3	_____	9	_____
4	_____	10	_____
5	_____	11	_____
6	_____	12	_____

Figure 14-8C in the textbook

Description:

_____

_____

_____

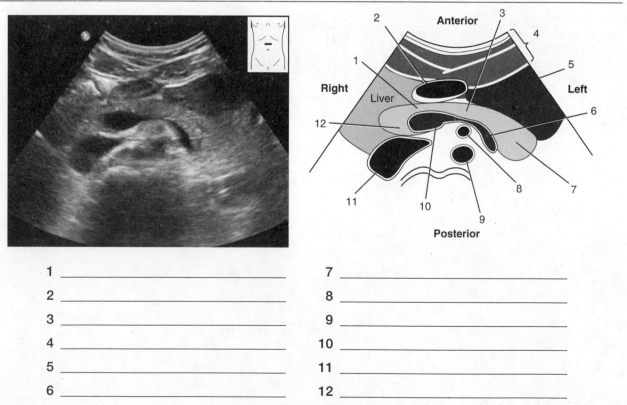

1	_____	7	_____
2	_____	8	_____
3	_____	9	_____
4	_____	10	_____
5	_____	11	_____
6	_____	12	_____

Figure 14-11 in the textbook

Description:

_____

_____

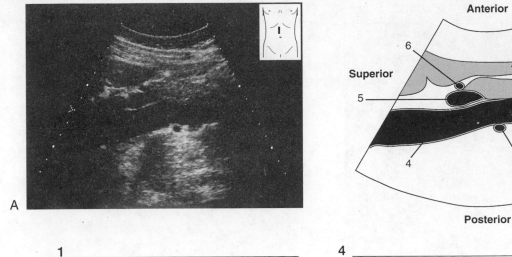

A

1	_____	4	_____
2	_____	5	_____
3	_____	6	_____

Figure 14-12A in the textbook

Description:

_____

_____

_____

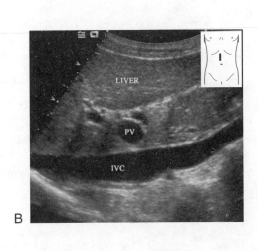

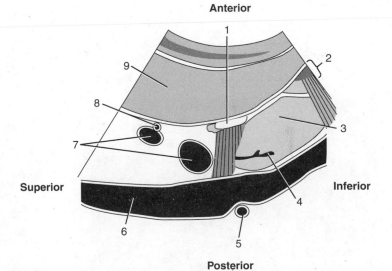

B

1	_____	6	_____
2	_____	7	_____
3	_____	8	_____
4	_____	9	_____
5	_____		

Figure 14-12B in the textbook

Description:

_____

_____

_____

125

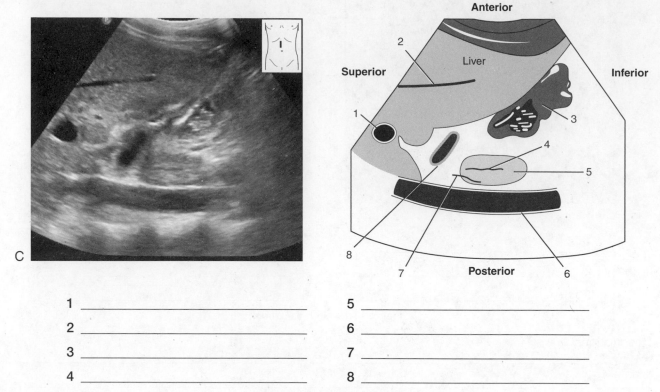

Figure 14-12C in the textbook

1	_____	5	_____
2	_____	6	_____
3	_____	7	_____
4	_____	8	_____

Description:

_____

_____

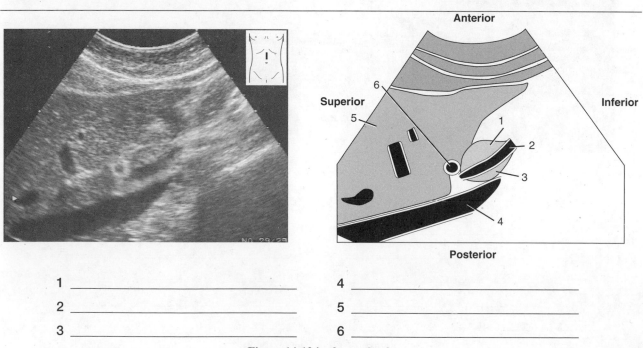

Figure 14-13 in the textbook

1	_____	4	_____
2	_____	5	_____
3	_____	6	_____

Description:

_____

_____

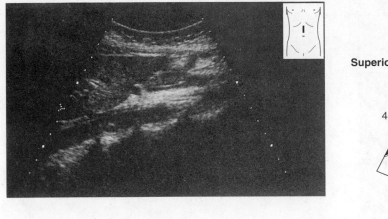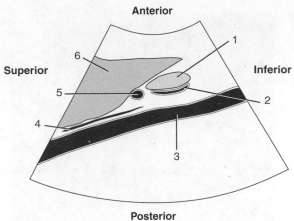

1	_____	4	_____
2	_____	5	_____
3	_____	6	_____

Figure 14-14 in the textbook

Description:

_____
_____
_____

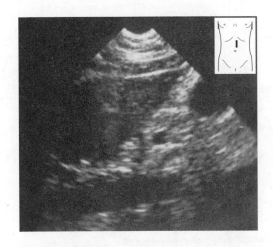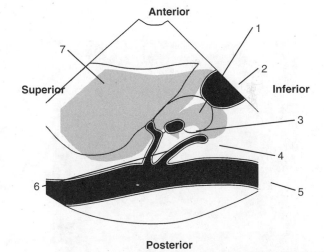

1	_____	5	_____
2	_____	6	_____
3	_____	7	_____
4	_____		

Figure 14-15 in the textbook

Description:

_____
_____
_____

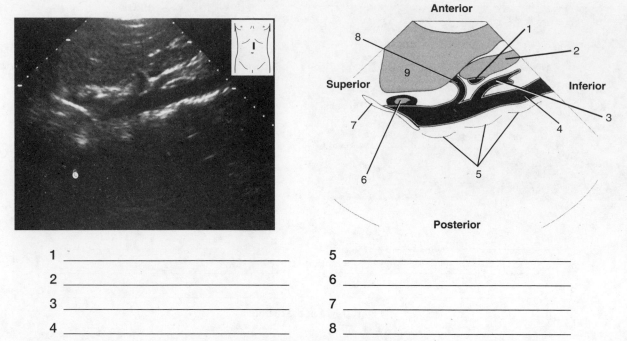

1 _____   5 _____

2 _____   6 _____

3 _____   7 _____

4 _____   8 _____

Figure 14-16 in the textbook

Description:

_____

_____

_____

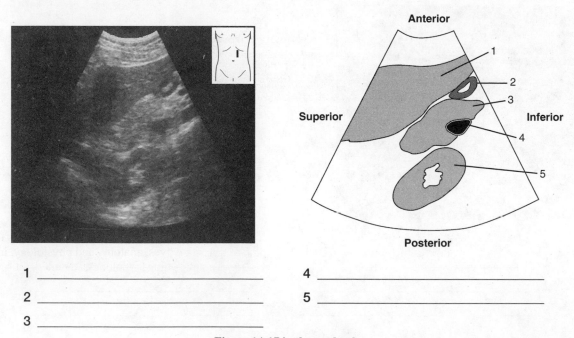

1 _____   4 _____

2 _____   5 _____

3 _____

Figure 14-17 in the textbook

Description:

_____

_____

_____

Chapter **14** **The Pancreas**

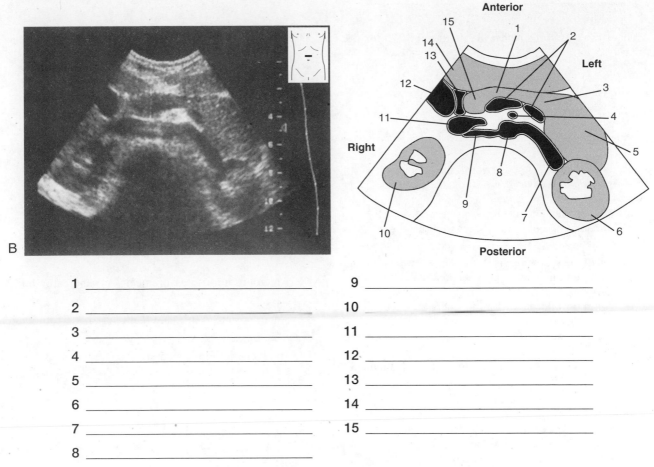

1 _____	9 _____
2 _____	10 _____
3 _____	11 _____
4 _____	12 _____
5 _____	13 _____
6 _____	14 _____
7 _____	15 _____
8 _____	

Figure 14-18B in the textbook

Description:

_____

_____

_____

V. CHAPTER SUBHEADINGS EXERCISE

1. Convert each chapter subheading into a question; for example, change "Gross Anatomy" to "What is the gross anatomy of the pancreas?" Write the answer to each question in a short paragraph in your notebook. Exchange answers with your lab partner and check each other's work. Refer back to the textbook for further information and explanation.

2. What questions do you still have about the chapter? Write your questions in your notebook.

VI. CHAPTER EVALUATION EXERCISE

Use a fresh sheet of notebook paper. Based on your work with the chapter and its accompanying laboratory assignments, identify three concepts you believe are the most important. You may draw from any of the assignments you have already completed in the previous pages including learning objectives, anatomy and physiology, images, or chapter subheadings. Include a detailed rationale in your answers.

Answer the questions below. Refer to page 370 for the answers.

Multiple Choice

1. The pancreas is shaped like the upside down letter
   a. H.
   b. N.
   c. U.
   d. C.

2. Which structures are posterior to the pancreas?
   a. Inferior vena cava (IVC), stomach, transverse colon
   b. IVC, diaphragm, aorta (AO)
   c. AO, stomach, duodenum
   d. Duodenum, connective prevertebral tissue, diaphragm

3. Which of the following structures enter the duodenum?
   a. Common bile duct, accessory pancreatic duct, duct of Wirsung
   b. Common bile duct, common hepatic duct, accessory pancreatic duct
   c. Common hepatic duct, cystic duct, main pancreatic duct
   d. Celiac duct, common hepatic duct, common bile duct

4. The body of the pancreas can best be described as lying anterior to
   a. superior mesenteric artery (SMA), splenic vein (SV), AO.
   b. SMA, SV, IVC.
   c. IMA, common bile duct (CBD), AO.
   d. inferior mesenteric artery (IMA), SV, IVC.

5. The tail of the pancreas can best be described as medial to the
   a. stomach.
   b. left kidney.
   c. splenic artery.
   d. splenic hilum.

Completion

Indicate the measurements of each of the following structures:

6. Anteroposterior measurement of pancreatic head _____

7. Anteroposterior measurement of pancreatic neck _____

8. Anteroposterior measurement of pancreatic body _____

9. Anteroposterior measurement of pancreatic tail _____

10. Total length of the pancreas _____

15 The Urinary and Adrenal Systems

I. MEMORIZATION EXERCISE

1. Write the key words in your notebook or on note cards. Write the words on one side of the notepaper and then write the definitions on the opposite side of the page or on the back of the paper. If using note cards, write the key word on the front and the definition on the back. *This step should be completed before the lab session begins.*

   Memorize the key word definitions silently for 5 minutes, then work with a lab partner and identify the words you still need help with. List the words here. Add additional rows if needed.

2. Next, write a short answer to the question just created.

   Example: "The nephron moves products from areas of high to low concentration by osmosis and active transport. It consists of Bowman's capsule, glomerulus, afferent and efferent arterioles, proximal and distal convoluted tubules, and collecting duct."

   Highlight or circle any part of your answers about which you are unsure, and check the answers in your textbook. If you are still unsure of the answers, put a question mark next to the answer(s) for the review session of the lab.

II. COMPREHENSION EXERCISE

1. Work with a lab partner to complete this exercise. You will need to write in your notebook. First, change each objective into a question.

   Example: "Explain the function of the nephron" becomes "What is the function of the nephron?"

III. APPLICATION OF ANATOMY AND PHYSIOLOGY EXERCISE

Directions to Students: Work on the following with your lab partner.
1. Label the parts of the urinary system.

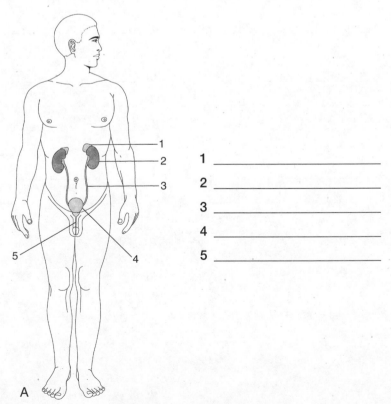

1 _____

2 _____

3 _____

4 _____

5 _____

Figure 15-1A in the textbook

2. Label the anterior view of kidneys and vasculature.

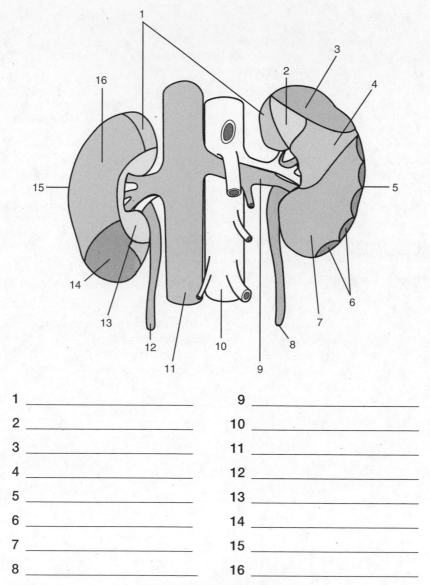

1	_____	9	_____
2	_____	10	_____
3	_____	11	_____
4	_____	12	_____
5	_____	13	_____
6	_____	14	_____
7	_____	15	_____
8	_____	16	_____

Figure 15-2 in the textbook

3. Label the posterior view of the kidneys and vasculature.

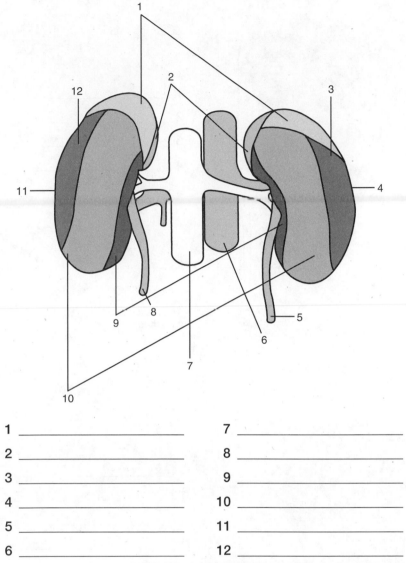

Figure 15-3 in the textbook

1	_____	7	_____
2	_____	8	_____
3	_____	9	_____
4	_____	10	_____
5	_____	11	_____
6	_____	12	_____

4. Label the layers surrounding the kidneys.

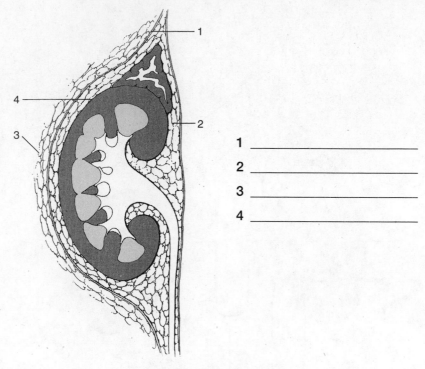

1 _____

2 _____

3 _____

4 _____

Figure 15-6 in the textbook

5. Label the internal kidney anatomy.

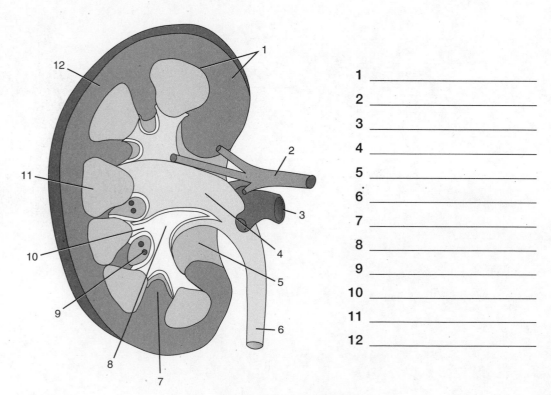

1 _____

2 _____

3 _____

4 _____

5 _____

6 _____

7 _____

8 _____

9 _____

10 _____

11 _____

12 _____

Figure 15-7 in the textbook

Chapter **15** **The Urinary and Adrenal Systems**

6. Label the cortical and juxtamedullary nephrons.

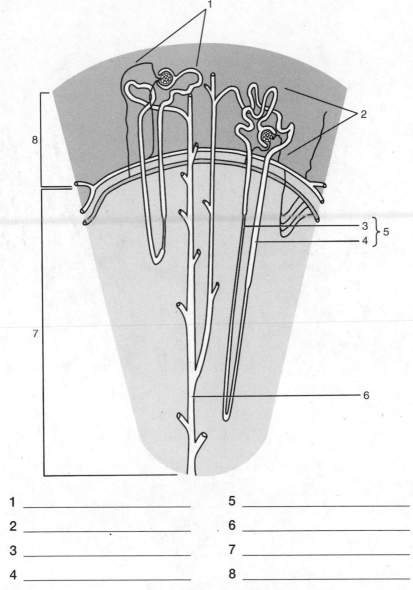

1 _____	5 _____
2 _____	6 _____
3 _____	7 _____
4 _____	8 _____

Figure 15-8 in the textbook

7. Label the nephron.

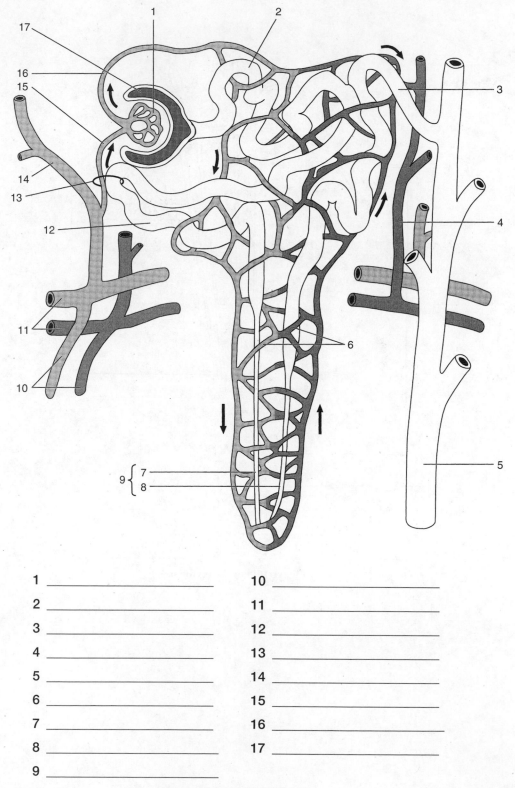

1 _____   10 _____

2 _____   11 _____

3 _____   12 _____

4 _____   13 _____

5 _____   14 _____

6 _____   15 _____

7 _____   16 _____

8 _____   17 _____

9 _____

Figure 15-12 in the textbook

8. Label the adrenal gland.

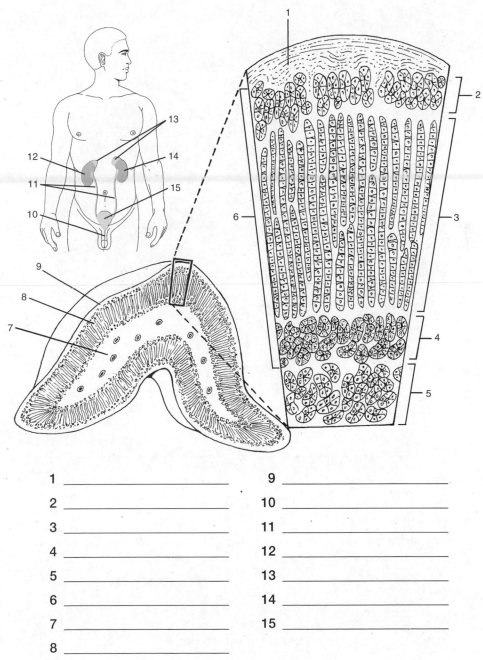

1	_____	9	_____
2	_____	10	_____
3	_____	11	_____
4	_____	12	_____
5	_____	13	_____
6	_____	14	_____
7	_____	15	_____
8	_____		

Figure 15-30 in the textbook

9. Label the adrenal vasculature.

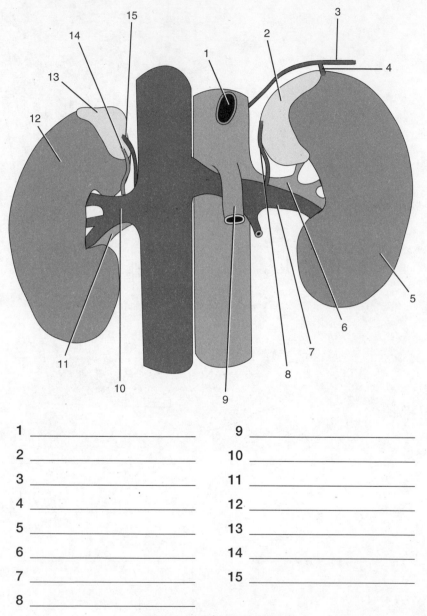

Figure 15-31 in the textbook

1 _____   9 _____
2 _____   10 _____
3 _____   11 _____
4 _____   12 _____
5 _____   13 _____
6 _____   14 _____
7 _____   15 _____
8 _____

10. Write two or three summary sentences on the physiology of the urinary and adrenal systems. Check your work against the physiology section of the textbook. What else can you add to your description?

_____

_____

_____

_____

_____

_____

_____

_____

_____

IV. IMAGE ANALYSIS EXERCISE

Work on the following figures with your lab partner. It's your choice! You can label all the sketches at once, then go back and label each image with your lab partner, or label an image and its accompanying sketch at the same time. Either way, the goal is to label correctly all of the sketches and carefully compare the sketch with the sonographic image.

For each sonographic image, write a brief observation that could be "presented" to your instructor, a clinical sonographer, or a sonologist. Please review the section from Chapter 1 on How to Describe Ultrasound Findings. Remember that you want to:

- **differentiate** abnormal echo patterns from normal echo patterns,
- **document** any differences in echo pattern appearance, and
- **describe** any difference in echo pattern appearance using sonographic terminology.

For each image, your assessment should include (1) the view of each major structure (axial or longitudinal; note: these are not the scanning planes) and (2) structures identified in the image with correct sonographic appearance description and measurements if shown.

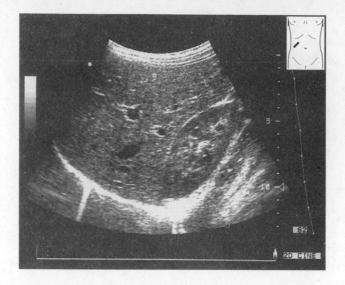 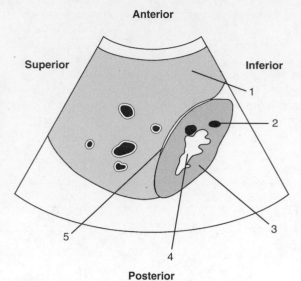

1 _____	4 _____
2 _____	5 _____
3 _____	

Figure 15-15 in the textbook

Description: _____

_____

_____

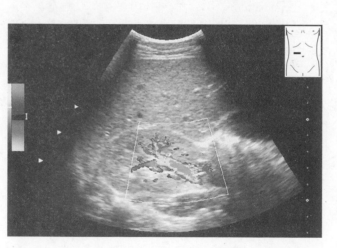 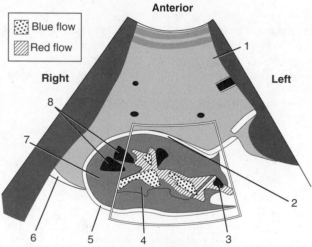

1 _____	5 _____
2 _____	6 _____
3 _____	7 _____
4 _____	8 _____

Figure 15-16 in the textbook

Description: _____

_____

_____

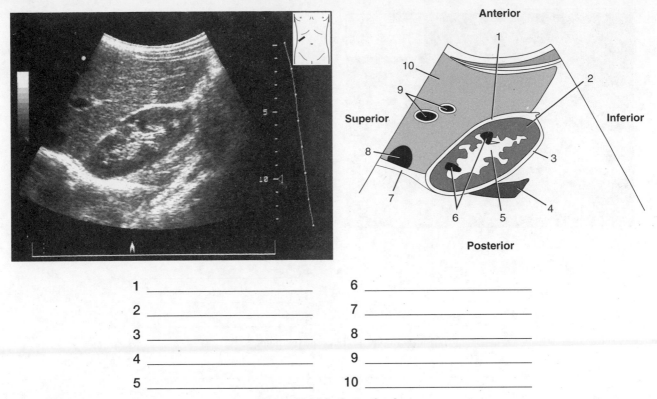

1 _____	6 _____
2 _____	7 _____
3 _____	8 _____
4 _____	9 _____
5 _____	10 _____

Figure 15-17 in the textbook

Description: _____

_____

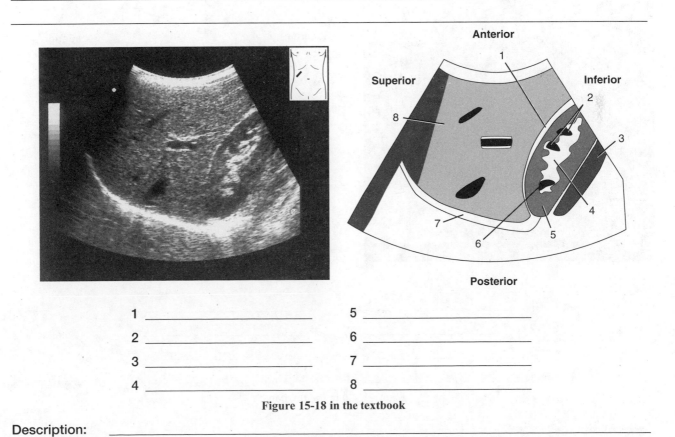

1 _____	5 _____
2 _____	6 _____
3 _____	7 _____
4 _____	8 _____

Figure 15-18 in the textbook

Description: _____

_____

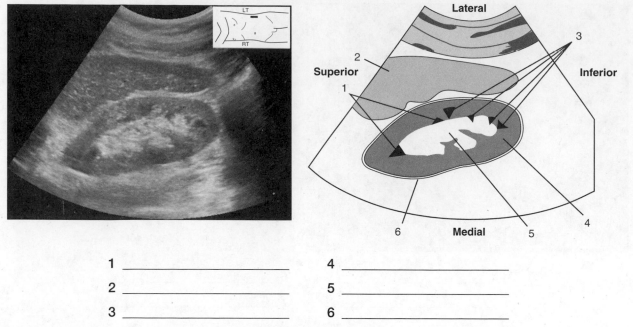

1	_____	4	_____
2	_____	5	_____
3	_____	6	_____

Figure 15-19 in the textbook

Description: _____

_____

_____

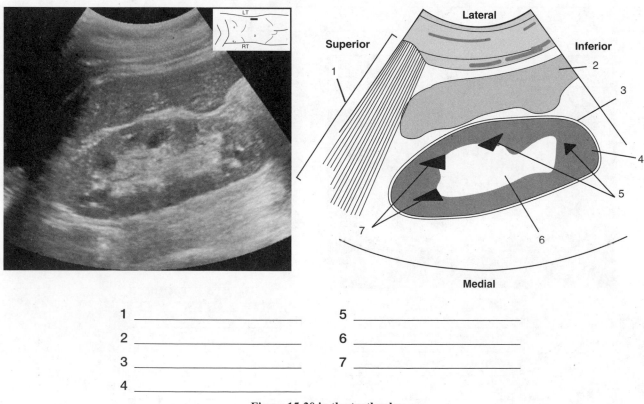

1	_____	5	_____
2	_____	6	_____
3	_____	7	_____
4	_____		

Figure 15-20 in the textbook

Description: _____

_____

_____

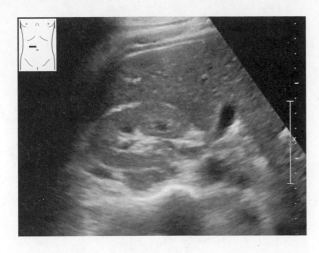

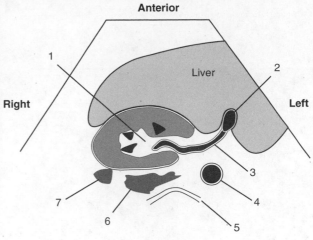

1 _____   5 _____

2 _____   6 _____

3 _____   7 _____

4 _____

Figure 15-21 in the textbook

Description: _____

_____

_____

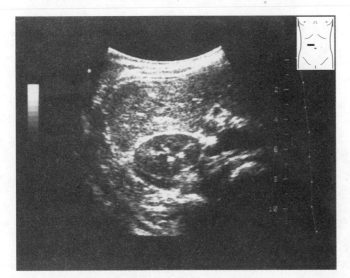

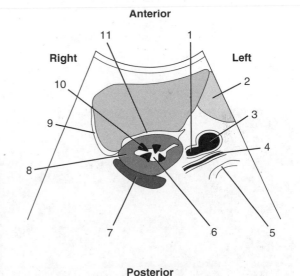

1 _____   7 _____

2 _____   8 _____

3 _____   9 _____

4 _____   10 _____

5 _____   11 _____

6 _____

Figure 15-22 in the textbook

Description: _____

_____

_____

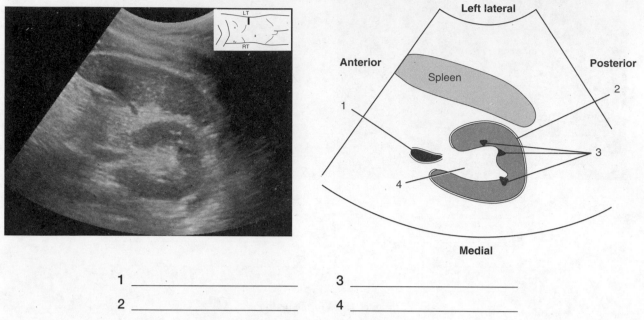

1 _____ 3 _____

2 _____ 4 _____

Figure 15-23 in the textbook

Description: _____

_____

_____

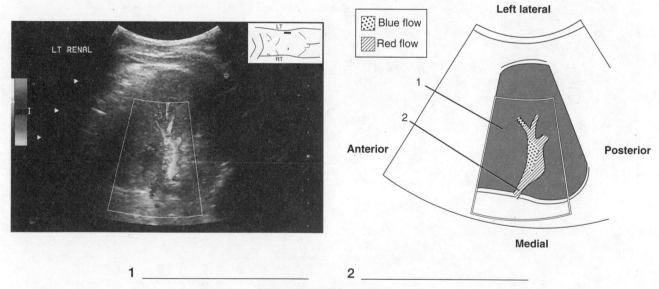

1 _____ 2 _____

Figure 15-24 in the textbook

Description: _____

_____

_____

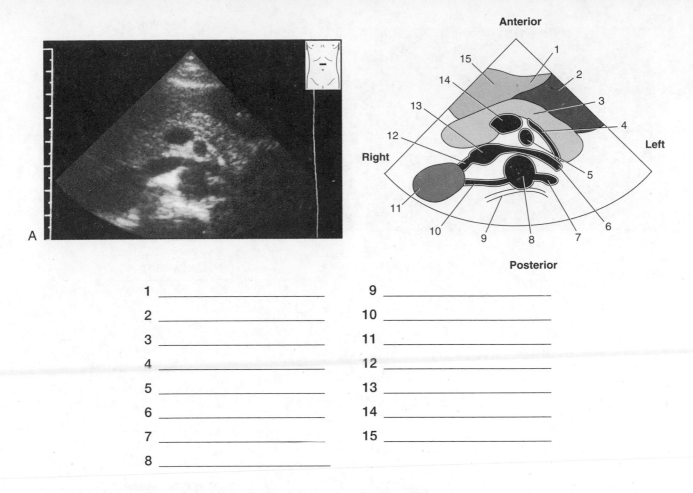

A

1 _____	9 _____
2 _____	10 _____
3 _____	11 _____
4 _____	12 _____
5 _____	13 _____
6 _____	14 _____
7 _____	15 _____
8 _____	

Figure 15-25A in the textbook

Description: _____

_____

_____

A

LONG RT KIDNEY MID (M)

Dist 9.62 cm
Dist 3.52 cm

1 _____	3 _____
2 _____	4 _____

Figure 15-26A in the textbook

Description: _____

_____

_____

145

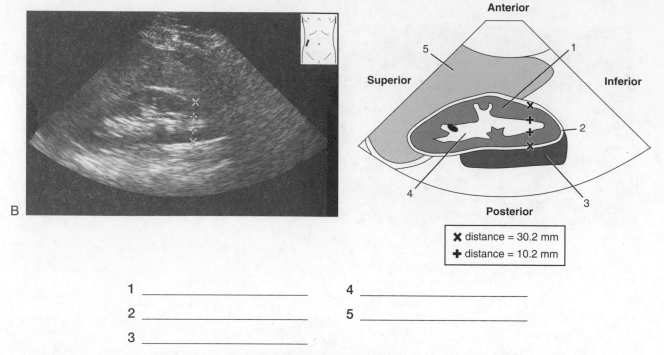

B

distance = 30.2 mm
distance = 10.2 mm

1 _____   4 _____
2 _____   5 _____
3 _____

Figure 15-26B in the textbook

Description: _____

_____

_____

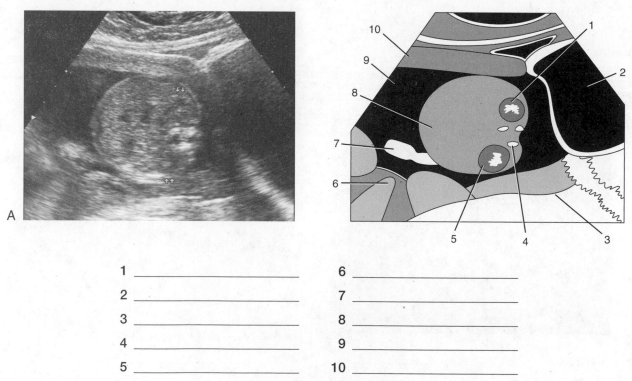

A

1 _____   6 _____
2 _____   7 _____
3 _____   8 _____
4 _____   9 _____
5 _____   10 _____

Figure 15-27A in the textbook

Description: _____

_____

_____

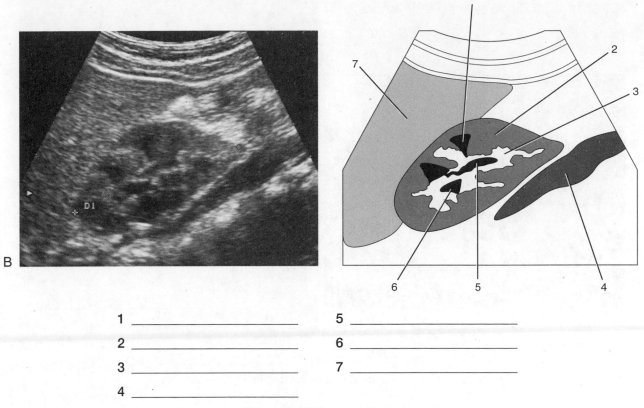

B

1	_____	5	_____
2	_____	6	_____
3	_____	7	_____
4	_____		

Figure 15-27B in the textbook

Description: _____

_____

_____

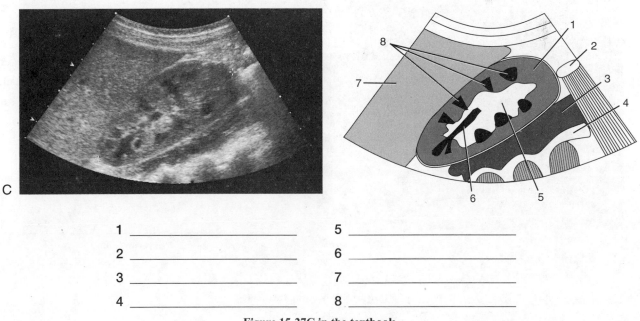

C

1	_____	5	_____
2	_____	6	_____
3	_____	7	_____
4	_____	8	_____

Figure 15-27C in the textbook

Description: _____

_____

_____

147

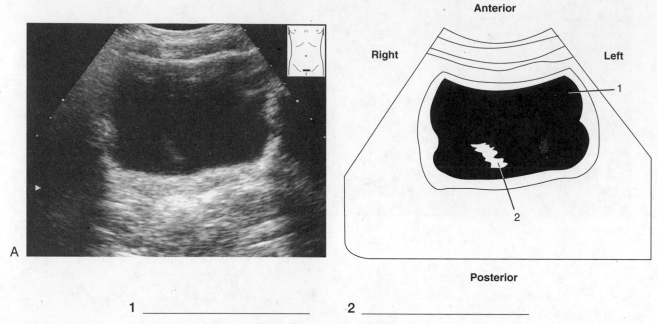

1 _____   2 _____

Figure 15-28A in the textbook

Description: _____

_____

_____

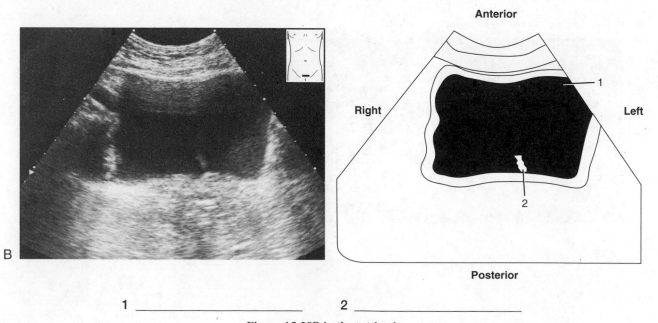

1 _____   2 _____

Figure 15-28B in the textbook

Description: _____

_____

_____

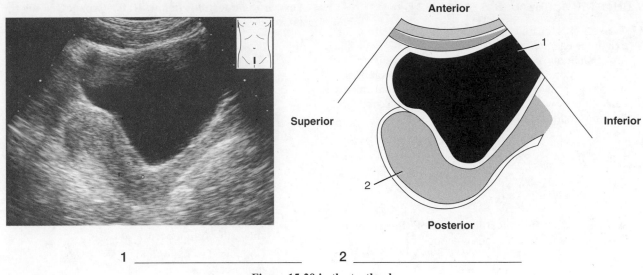

1 _____ 2 _____

Figure 15-29 in the textbook

Description: _____

_____

_____

V. CHAPTER SUBHEADINGS EXERCISE

1. Convert each chapter subheading into a question; for example, change "Gross Anatomy" to "What is the gross anatomy of the kidney?" Write the answer to each question in a short paragraph in your notebook. Exchange answers with your lab partner and check each other's work. Refer back to the textbook for further information and explanation.

2. What questions do you still have about the chapter? Write your questions in your notebook.

VI. CHAPTER EVALUATION EXERCISE

Use a fresh sheet of notebook paper. Based on your work with the chapter and its accompanying laboratory assignments, identify three concepts you believe are the most important. You may draw from any of the assignments you have already completed in the previous pages including learning objectives, anatomy and physiology, images, or chapter subheadings. Include a detailed rationale in your answers.

Answer the questions below. Refer to page 370 for the answers.

Matching

1. ___ Location where the renal artery enters.
2. ___ Central area of the kidney that houses the renal vessels, nerves, and lymphatics.
3. ___ Contains the renal corpuscle and proximal and distal convoluted tubules of the nephron.
4. ___ Area where filtration and reabsorption occur.
5. ___ Composed of major and minor calyces.
6. ___ Upper expanded end of the ureter.

a. Renal cortex
b. Renal sinus
c. Renal medulla
d. Renal hilum
e. Infundibulum
f. Renal pelvis

True/False

7. The female urethra is longer than the male urethra.
8. The adrenal gland is easily visualized sonographically in neonates.
9. The kidneys are intraperitoneal in location.
10. At birth, the adrenal glands are one-half the size of the kidneys but then rapidly shrink.

16 Abdominal Vasculature

I. MEMORIZATION EXERCISE

Write the key words in your notebook or on note cards. Write the words on one side of the notepaper and then write the definitions on the opposite side of the page or on the back of the paper. If using note cards, write the key word on the front and the definition on the back. *This step should be completed before the lab session begins.*

Memorize the key word definitions silently for 5 minutes, then work with a lab partner and identify the words you still need help with. List the words here. Add additional rows if needed.

II. COMPREHENSION EXERCISE

1. Work with a lab partner to complete this exercise. You will need to write in your notebook. First, change each objective into a question.

   Example: "Review abdominal arterial and venous anatomy and sonographic appearance" becomes "What is the abdominal arterial and venous anatomy?"

2. Next, write a short answer to the question just created. You can divide the answer into parts.

   Example: "Abdominal arterial anatomy consists of aorta, celiac artery, superior and inferior mesenteric arteries, and the renal arteries, with average diameter ranging from 0.30 cm (IMA) to 2.0-2.5 cm (aorta). Abdominal venous anatomy consists of inferior vena cava, renal veins, hepatic veins, superior mesenteric vein, splenic and portal veins with average diameter ranging from 0.40 cm (hepatic and splenic veins) to 2.5-3.0 cm (IVC)."

   Highlight or circle any part of your answers about which you are unsure, and check the answers in your textbook. If you are still unsure of the answers, put a question mark next to the answer(s) for the review session of the lab.

1. Label the abdominal vasculature and as many branches as you can from memory. Include each vessel's orientation in the body (either vertical, horizontal, vertical oblique, or horizontal oblique). Ask your lab partner to critique your work. What did you miss? Check your drawing using Figure 16.1 in your textbook and complete any missing labels. Below the diagram, write two or three summary sentences of the physiology of the arterial and venous vasculature. Ask your lab partner to check your work. Now check your work against the physiology section in the textbook. What else can you add to your description?

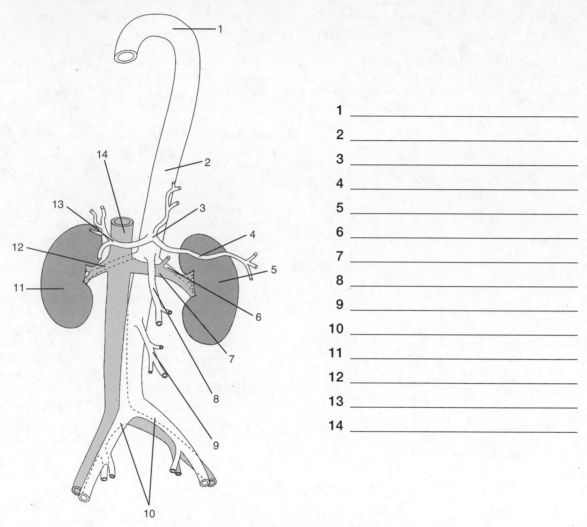

1 _____

2 _____

3 _____

4 _____

5 _____

6 _____

7 _____

8 _____

9 _____

10 _____

11 _____

12 _____

13 _____

14 _____

Figure 16-1 in the textbook

Description:

_____

_____

_____

IV. IMAGE ANALYSIS EXERCISE

Work on the following figures with your lab partner. It's your choice! You can label all the sketches at once, then go back and label each image with your lab partner, or label an image and its accompanying sketch at the same time. Either way, the goal is to label correctly all of the sketches and carefully compare the sketch with the sonographic image.

For each sonographic image, write a brief observation that could be "presented" to your instructor, a clinical sonographer, or a sonologist. Please review the section from Chapter 1 on How to Describe Ultrasound Findings. Remember that you want to:

- **differentiate** abnormal echo patterns from normal echo patterns,
- **document** any differences in echo pattern appearance, and
- **describe** any difference in echo pattern appearance using sonographic terminology.

For each image, your assessment should include (1) the view of each major structure (axial or longitudinal; note: these are not the scanning planes) and (2) structures identified in the image with correct sonographic appearance description and measurements if shown.

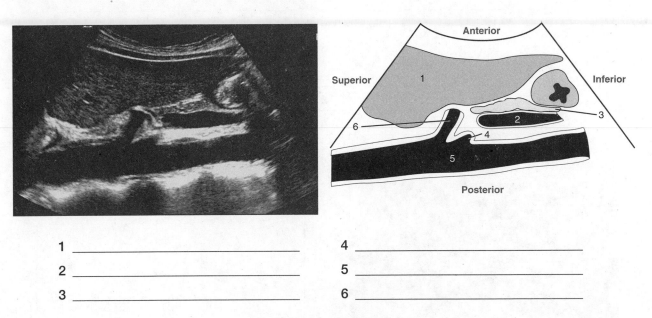

1 _____   4 _____

2 _____   5 _____

3 _____   6 _____

Figure 16-2 in the textbook

Description:

_____

_____

_____

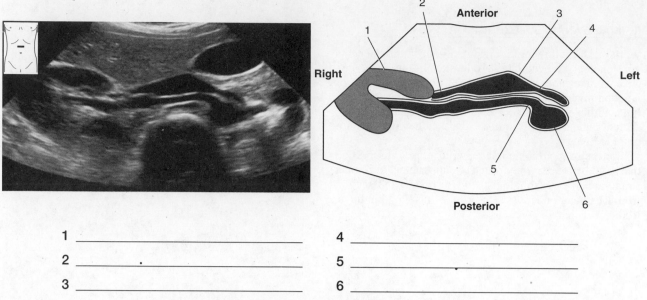

1	_____	4	_____
2	_____	5	_____
3	_____	6	_____

Figure 16-3 in the textbook

Description:

_____

_____

_____

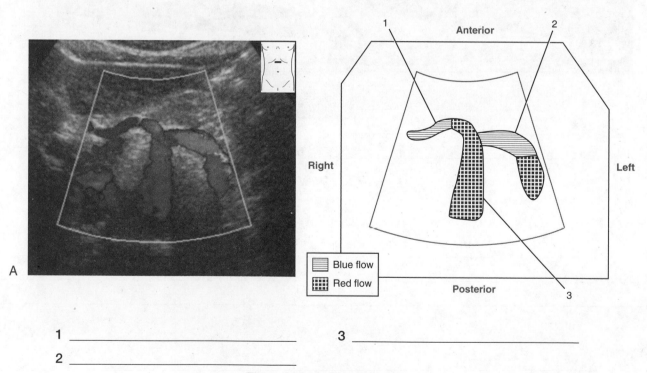

| 1 | _____ | 3 | _____ |
| 2 | _____ | | |

Figure 16-8A in the textbook

Description:

_____

_____

_____

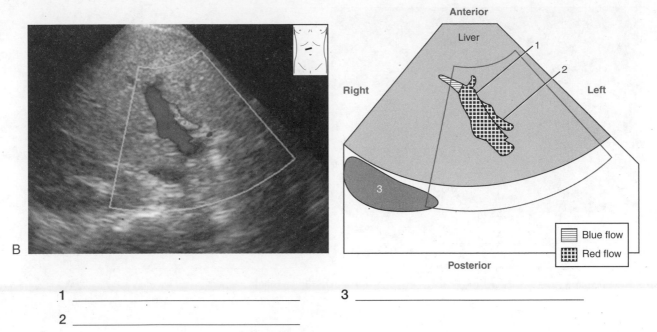

1 _____ 3 _____
2 _____

Figure 16-8B in the textbook

Description:

_____

_____

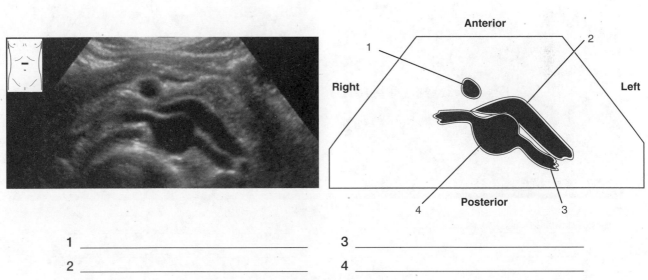

1 _____ 3 _____
2 _____ 4 _____

Figure 16-14 in the textbook

Description:

_____

_____

_____

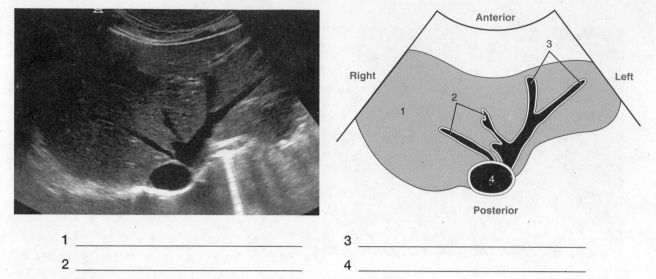

| 1 | _____ | 3 | _____ |
| 2 | _____ | 4 | _____ |

Figure 16-15 in the textbook

Description:

_____

_____

_____

1	_____	4	_____
2	_____	5	_____
3	_____		

Figure 16-16 in the textbook

Description:

_____

_____

_____

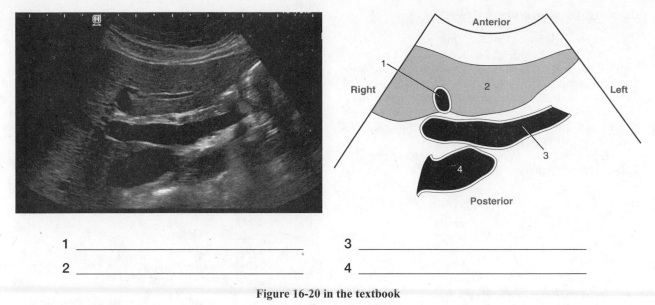

1 _____	3 _____
2 _____	4 _____

Figure 16-20 in the textbook

Description:

_____

_____

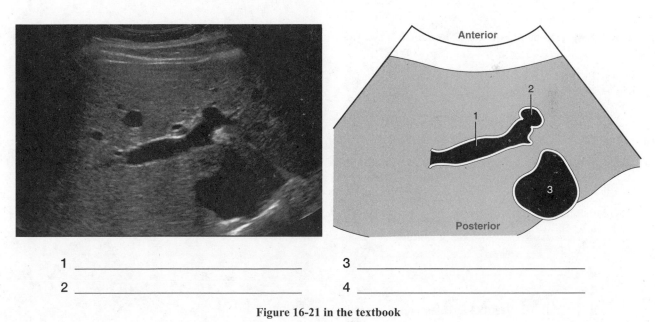

1 _____	3 _____
2 _____	4 _____

Figure 16-21 in the textbook

Description:

_____

_____

_____

V. CHAPTER SUBHEADINGS EXERCISE

1. Convert each chapter subheading into a question; for example, change "Sonographic Appearance" to "What is the sonographic appearance of the arterial and venous vessels?" Briefly write the answer to each question in a short paragraph in your notebook. Exchange answers with your lab partner and check each other's work. Refer back to the textbook for further information and explanation.
2. What questions do you still have about the chapter? Write your questions in your notebook.

VI. CHAPTER EVALUATION EXERCISE

Use a fresh sheet of notebook paper. Based on your work with the chapter and its accompanying laboratory assignments, identify three concepts you believe are the most important. You may draw from any of the assignments you have already completed in the previous pages including learning objectives, anatomy and physiology, images, or chapter subheadings. Include a detailed rationale in your answers.

Answer the questions below. Refer to page 371 for the answers.

Multiple Choice

1. What is the most common anatomic variant of the abdominal arterial vessels?
   a. Replaced right hepatic artery
   b. Duplicated renal artery
   c. Common origin of the celiac artery and SMA
   d. Duplication of the common hepatic artery

2. Which fluid dynamic theory is used to determine *volumetric* flow?
   a. Bernoulli's
   b. Poiseuille's
   c. Ohm's
   d. Doppler

3. Which variable creates the greatest resistance to flow?
   a. Length
   b. Viscosity
   c. Radius
   d. Pressure gradient

4. What is the key factor that determines the blood distribution throughout the body?
   a. Metabolic need of a tissue or organ
   b. Cardiac stroke volume
   c. Cardiac output
   d. Velocity of blood flow

5. What is considered the resistive component of the arterial system?
   a. Conducting vessels
   b. Capillaries
   c. Distributing vessels
   d. Arterioles

6. Bernoulli's equation demonstrates the relationship between
   a. pressure and velocity.
   b. radius and resistance.
   c. viscosity and lumen size.
   d. volume and resistance.

7. Ohm's law is used to demonstrate the relationship of
   a. pressure and velocity.
   b. volume and resistance.
   c. viscosity and lumen size.
   d. radius and resistance.

8. Which imaging modality supplies quantitative data on a blood vessel?
   a. Color Doppler
   b. 2D gray scale
   c. Power Doppler
   d. Pulsed wave Doppler

9. What part of the spectral Doppler waveform demonstrates downstream resistance to flow?
   a. Systolic peak
   b. Systolic window
   c. Diastolic flow
   d. Spectral broadening

10. A spectral waveform from a low resistive vessel will have
   a. minimal or absent diastolic flow.
   b. elevated peak systolic velocity.
   c. reverse flow in diastole.
   d. constant forward flow in diastole.

17 The Spleen

I. MEMORIZATION EXERCISE

1. Write the key words in your notebook or on note cards. Write the words on one side of the notepaper and then write the definitions on the opposite side of the page or on the back of the paper. If using note cards, write the key word on the front and the definition on the back. *This step should be completed before the lab session begins.*

   Memorize the key word definitions silently for 5 minutes, then work with a lab partner and identify the words you still need help with. List the words here. Add additional rows if needed.

II. COMPREHENSION EXERCISE

1. Work with a lab partner to complete this exercise. You will need to write in your notebook. First, change each objective into a question.

   Example: "Describe the location of the spleen" becomes "What is the location of the spleen?"

2. Next, write a short answer to the question just created.

   Example: "The spleen is in the left hypochondrium. It lies posterior and lateral to the stomach fundus and body, tail of the pancreas, and left colic flexure."

Highlight or circle any part of your answers about which you are unsure, and check the answers in your textbook. If you are still unsure of the answers, put a question mark next to the answer(s) for the review session of the lab.

III. APPLICATION OF ANATOMY AND PHYSIOLOGY EXERCISE

1. Label the spleen and its vasculature.

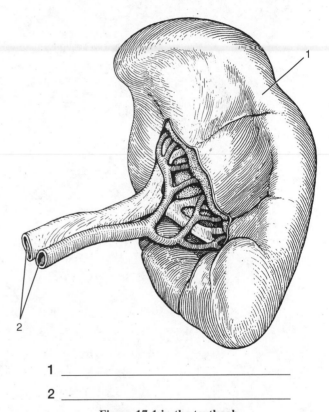

1 _____

2 _____

Figure 17-1 in the textbook

2. Label each dimension and structure shown in the diagram.

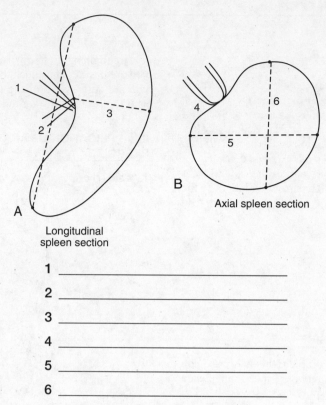

A

Longitudinal
spleen section

B

Axial spleen section

1 _____

2 _____

3 _____

4 _____

5 _____

6 _____

Figure 17-3A and B in the textbook

3. Label the splenic artery and surrounding structures.

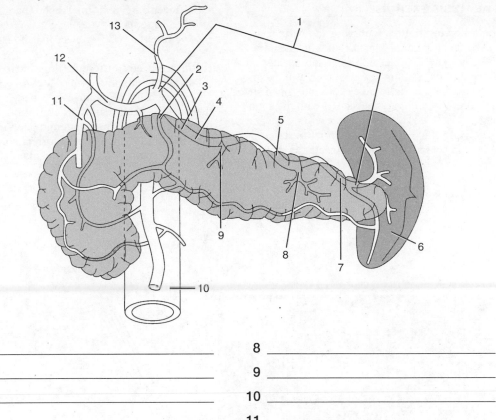

1 _____   8 _____

2 _____   9 _____

3 _____   10 _____

4 _____   11 _____

5 _____   12 _____

6 _____   13 _____

7 _____

Figure 17-4 in the textbook

4. Write two or three summary sentences on the physiology of the spleen. Check your work against the physiology section of the textbook. What else can you add to your description?

_____

_____

_____

IV. IMAGE ANALYSIS EXERCISE

Work on the following figures with your lab partner. It's your choice! You can label all the sketches at once, then go back and label each image with your lab partner, or label an image and its accompanying sketch at the same time. Either way, the goal is to label correctly all of the sketches and carefully compare the sketch with the sonographic image.

For each sonographic image, write a brief observation that could be "presented" to your instructor, a clinical sonographer, or a sonologist. Please review the section from Chapter 1 on How to Describe Ultrasound Findings. Remember that you want to:

- **differentiate** abnormal echo patterns from normal echo patterns,
- **document** any differences in echo pattern appearance, and
- **describe** any difference in echo pattern appearance using sonographic terminology.

For each image, your assessment should include (1) the view of each major structure (axial or longitudinal; note: these are not the scanning planes) and (2) structures identified in the image with correct sonographic appearance description and measurements if shown.

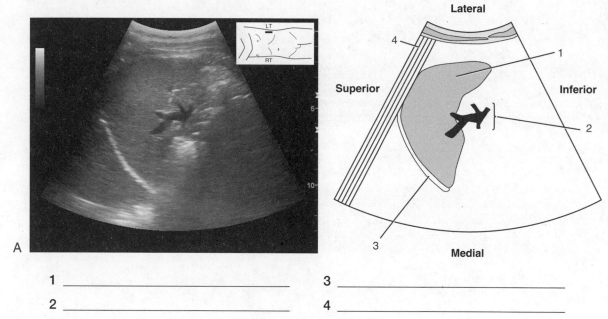

1 _____   3 _____

2 _____   4 _____

Figure 17-6A in the textbook

Description: _____
_____
_____

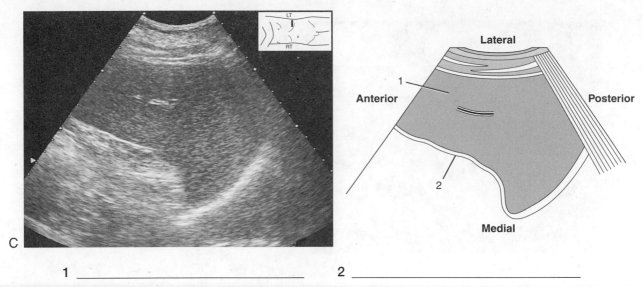

C

1 _____ 2 _____

Figure 17-6C in the textbook

Description: _____
_____
_____

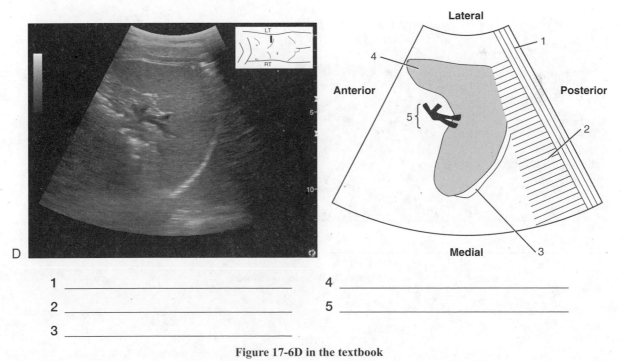

D

1 _____ 4 _____

2 _____ 5 _____

3 _____

Figure 17-6D in the textbook

Description: _____
_____
_____

163

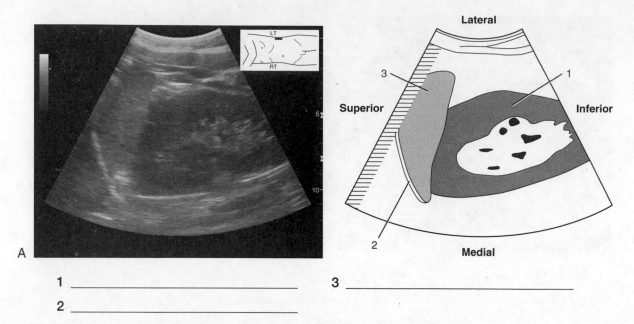

A

1 _____   3 _____

2 _____

Figure 17-7A in the textbook

Description: _____

_____

_____

B

1 _____   2 _____

Figure 17-7B in the textbook

Description: _____

_____

_____

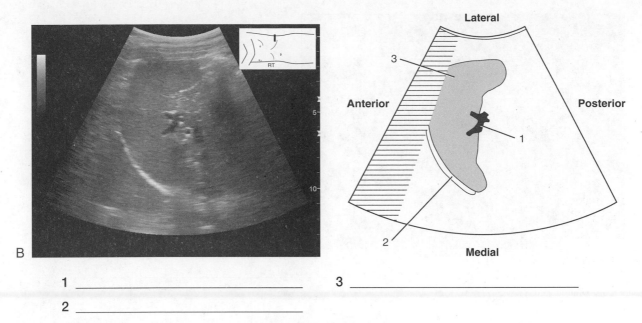

B

1 _____   3 _____

2 _____

Figure 17-8B in the textbook

Description: _____

_____

_____

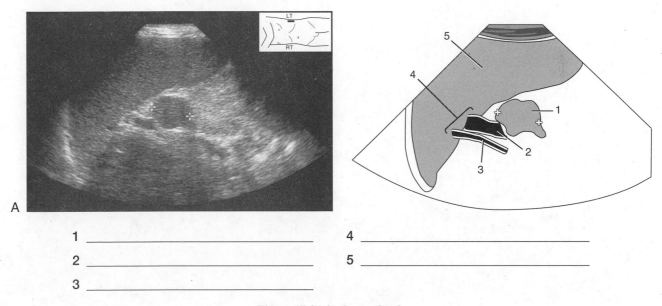

A

1 _____   4 _____

2 _____   5 _____

3 _____

Figure 17-9A in the textbook

Description: _____

_____

_____

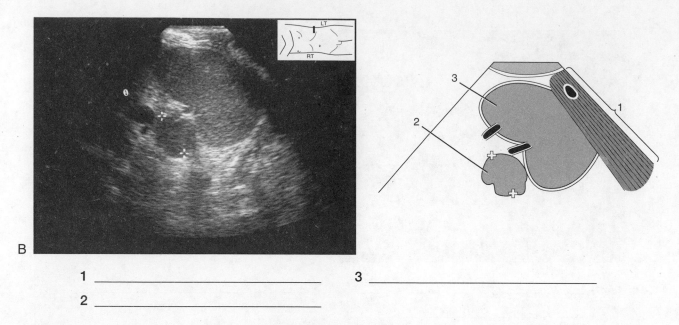

B

1 _____   3 _____

2 _____

Figure 17-9B in the textbook

Description: _____

_____

_____

V. CHAPTER SUBHEADINGS EXERCISE

1. Convert each chapter subheading into a question; for example, change "Gross Anatomy" to "What is the gross anatomy of the spleen?" Write the answer to each question in a short paragraph in your notebook. Exchange answers with your lab partner and check each other's work. Refer back to the textbook for further information and explanations.

2. What questions do you still have about the chapter? Write your questions in your notebook.

VI. CHAPTER EVALUATION EXERCISE

Use a fresh sheet of notebook paper. Based on your work with the chapter and its accompanying laboratory assignments, identify three concepts you believe are the most important. You may draw from any of the assignments you've already completed in the previous pages including learning objectives, anatomy and physiology, images, or chapter subheadings. Include a detailed rationale in your answers.

Answer the questions below. Refer to page 371 for the answers.

Multiple Choice

1. The splenic vein conveys venous blood from the spleen and courses along the gastrolienal ligament to its confluence with the
   a. superior mesenteric artery.
   b. splenic artery.
   c. superior mesenteric vein.
   d. main portal vein.

2. All of the following are functions of the spleen except:
   a. Defense
   b. Hematopoiesis
   c. Serves as a blood reservoir
   d. Stores bile

Matching

___ 3. The process of removing abnormal red blood cells by the spleen	a. Erythrocyte
___ 4. Oxygen-carrying and iron-containing pigment of red blood cells	b. Phagocytosis
___ 5. The process that produces erythrocytes and white blood cells in the developing fetus	c. Hematopoiesis
___ 6. The term for a red blood cell	d. White pulp
___ 7. The process of removing nuclei from old red blood cells	e. Culling
___ 8. Responsible for phagocytosis of damaged or old cells	f. Hemoglobin
___ 9. Found in the spleen, consists of lymphatic tissue, and is where immune functions take place	g. Reticuloendothelial system
___ 10. The process of removing worn-out and abnormal red blood cells and platelets from the bloodstream by phagocyte cells in the spleen	h. Pitting

The Gastrointestinal System 18

I. MEMORIZATION EXERCISE

1. Write the key words in your notebook or on note cards. Write the words on one side of the notepaper and then write the definitions on the opposite side of the page or on the back of the paper. If using note cards, write the key word on the front and the definition on the back. *This step should be completed before the lab session begins.*

   Memorize the key word definitions silently for 5 minutes, then work with a lab partner and identify the words you still need help with. List the words here. Add additional rows if needed.

II. COMPREHENSION EXERCISE

1. Work with a lab partner to complete this exercise. You will need to write in your notebook. First, change each objective into a question.

   Example: "Identify the five principal layers of bowel, known as the gut signature"

becomes *"What are the five principal layers of bowel, known as the gut signature?"*

2. Next, write a short answer to the question just created.

   Example: "The five layers of bowel, from the inside out, are the innermost layer, the mucosa, which is in contact with the intestinal contents; next is the submucosa; the muscular layer, muscularis; serosa; and the outermost layer, mesothelium, which covers the bowel loops."

Highlight or circle any part of your answers about which you are unsure and check the answers in your textbook. If you are still unsure of the answers, put a question mark next to the answer(s) for the review session of the lab.

168

III. APPLICATION OF ANATOMY AND PHYSIOLOGY EXERCISE

1. Label the parts of the GI tract.

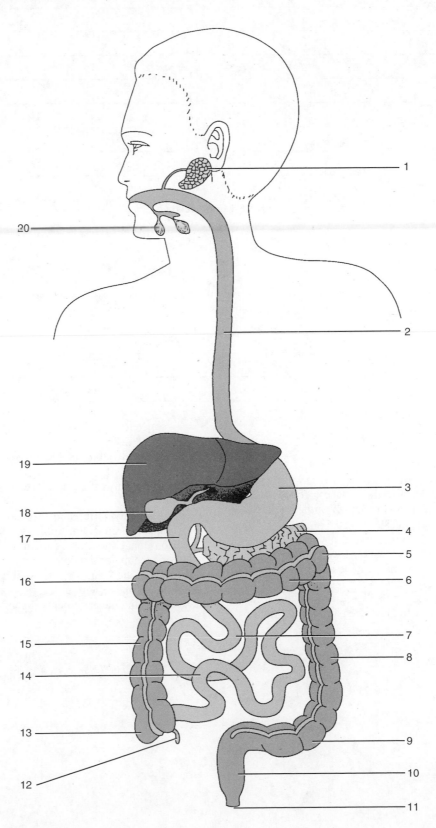

1 _____   11 _____

2 _____   12 _____

3 _____   13 _____

4 _____   14 _____

5 _____   15 _____

6 _____   16 _____

7 _____   17 _____

8 _____   18 _____

9 _____   19 _____

10 _____   20 _____

Figure 18-1 in the textbook.

2. Write two or three summary sentences on the physiology of the GI tract. Now check your work against the physiology section in the textbook. What else can you add to your description?

_____

_____

_____

IV. IMAGE ANALYSIS EXERCISE

Work on the following figures with your lab partner. It's your choice! You can label all the sketches at once, then go back and label each image with your lab partner, or label an image and its accompanying sketch at the same time. Either way, the goal is to label correctly all of the sketches and carefully compare the sketch with the sonographic image.

For each sonographic image, write a brief observation that could be "presented" to your instructor, a clinical sonographer, or a sonologist. Please review the section from Chapter 1 on How to Describe Ultrasound Findings. Remember that you want to:

- **differentiate** abnormal echo patterns from normal echo patterns,
- **document** any differences in echo pattern appearance, and
- **describe** any difference in echo pattern appearance using sonographic terminology.

For each image, your assessment should include (1) the view of each major structure (axial or longitudinal; note: these are not the scanning planes) and (2) structures identified in the image with correct sonographic appearance description and measurements if shown.

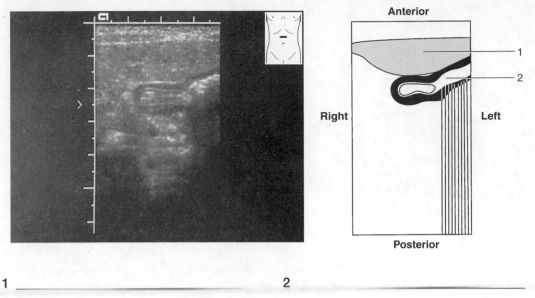

Figure 18-3 in the textbook

Description: _____

_____

_____

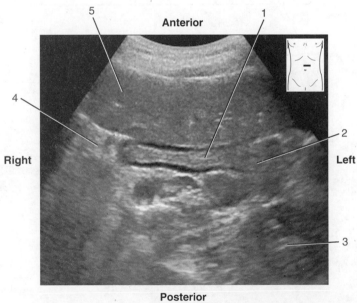

1 _____   4 _____

2 _____   5 _____

3 _____

Figure 18-4 in the textbook

Description: _____

_____

_____

Chapter **18** **The Gastrointestinal System**

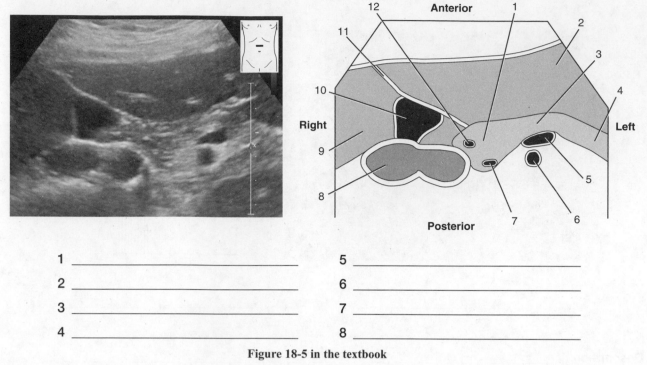

1	_____	5	_____
2	_____	6	_____
3	_____	7	_____
4	_____	8	_____

Figure 18-5 in the textbook

Description: _____

_____

_____

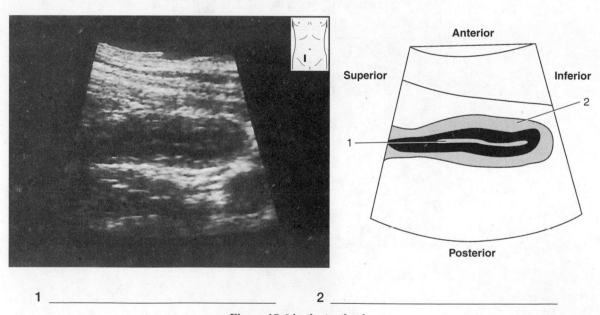

| 1 | _____ | 2 | _____ |

Figure 18-6 in the textbook

Description: _____

_____

_____

Chapter **18**   **The Gastrointestinal System**

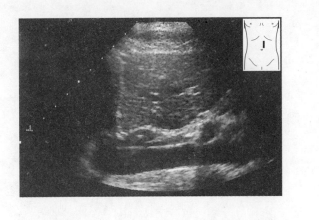

1 _____   4 _____

2 _____   5 _____

3 _____   6 _____

Figure 18-10 in the textbook

Description _____

_____

_____

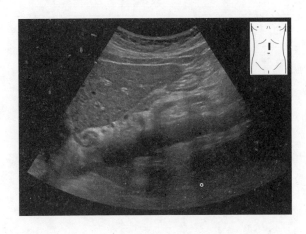

1 _____   4 _____

2 _____   5 _____

3 _____   6 _____

Figure 18-11 in the textbook

Description _____

_____

_____

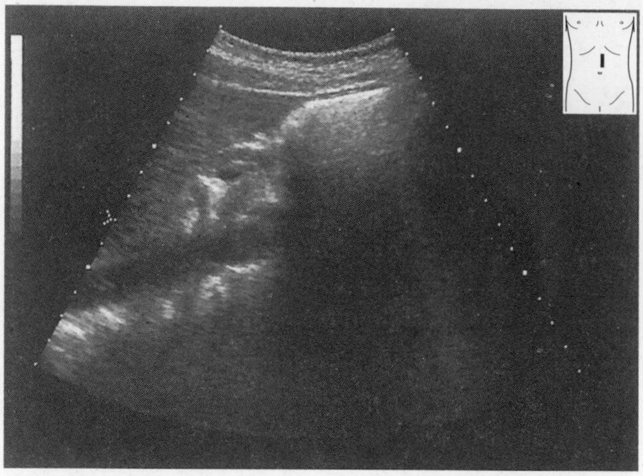

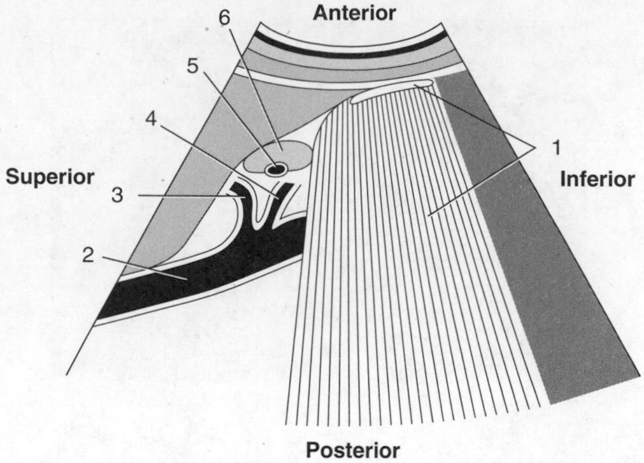

1 _____	4 _____
2 _____	5 _____
3 _____	6 _____

Figure 18-13 in the textbook

Description: _____

_____

_____

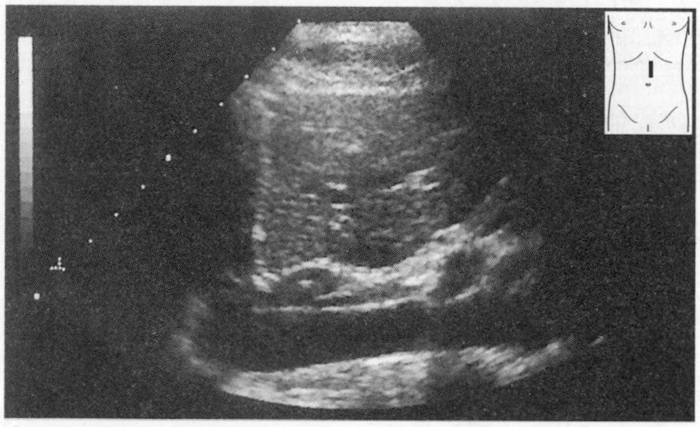

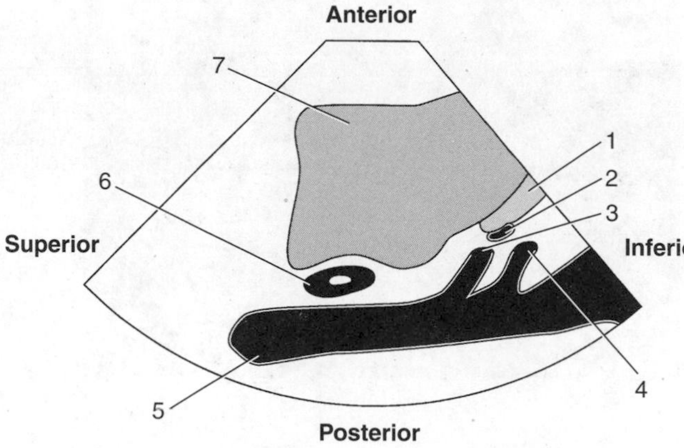

1 _____	5 _____
2 _____	6 _____
3 _____	7 _____
4 _____	

Figure 18-15 in the textbook

Description: _____

_____

_____

174

Chapter **18   The Gastrointestinal System**

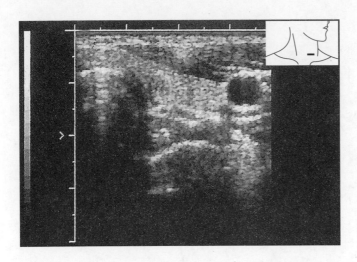
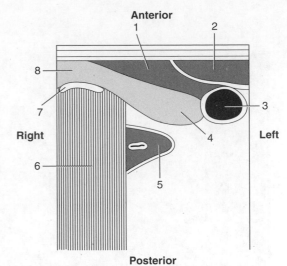

1 _____ 5 _____

2 _____ 6 _____

3 _____ 7 _____

4 _____ 8 _____

Figure 18-16 in the textbook

Description: _____

_____

_____

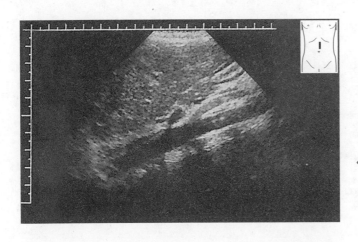

1 _____ 6 _____

2 _____ 7 _____

3 _____ 8 _____

4 _____ 9 _____

5 _____ 10 _____

Figure 18-17 in the textbook

Description: _____

_____

_____

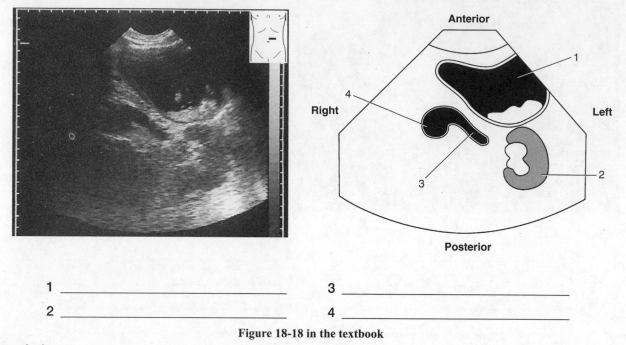

1 _____ 3 _____

2 _____ 4 _____

Figure 18-18 in the textbook

Description: _____
_____
_____

1 _____ 5 _____

2 _____ 6 _____

3 _____ 7 _____

4 _____ 8 _____

Figure 18-19 in the textbook

Description: _____
_____
_____

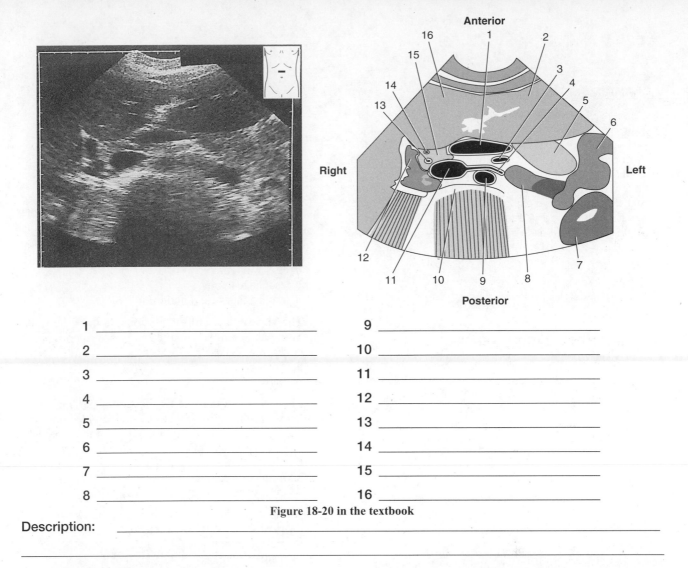

Anterior

Right   Left

Posterior

1 _____	9 _____
2 _____	10 _____
3 _____	11 _____
4 _____	12 _____
5 _____	13 _____
6 _____	14 _____
7 _____	15 _____
8 _____	16 _____

Figure 18-20 in the textbook

Description: _____

_____

_____

Anterior

Right   Left

Posterior

1 _____	3 _____
2 _____	4 _____

Figure 18-25 in the textbook

Description: _____

_____

_____

V. CHAPTER SUBHEADINGS EXERCISE

1. Convert each chapter subheading into a question; for example, change "Gross Anatomy" to "What is the gross anatomy of the GI tract?" Write the answer to each question in a short paragraph in your notebook. Exchange answers with your lab partner and check each other's work. Refer back to the textbook for further information and explanations.
2. What questions do you still have about the chapter? Write your questions in your notebook.

VI. CHAPTER EVALUATION EXERCISE

Use a fresh sheet of notebook paper. Based on your work with the chapter and its accompanying laboratory assignments, identify three concepts you believe are the most important. You may draw from any of the assignments you've already completed in the previous pages including learning objectives, anatomy and physiology, images, or chapter subheadings. Include a detailed rationale in your answers.

Answer the questions below. Refer to page 371 for the answers.

Multiple Choice

1. Another name for the gastrointestinal tract is the
   a. parenteral canal.
   b. alimentary canal.
   c. mucosal canal.
   d. mediastinum.

2. The characteristic appearance of the bowel wall can be described by a term known as the
   a. omentum.
   b. haustra.
   c. gut signature.
   d. mesentery.

3. The parietal peritoneum covers the anterior, lateral and posterior walls of the abdominopelvic cavity and forms a closed sac.
   a. True
   b. False

5. The deepest fold of the peritoneal cavity in females is called the
   a. rectouterine pouch.
   b. posterior cul-de-sac.
   c. pouch of Douglas.
   d. All are correct.
   e. None are correct.

6. The esophagus is a part of the GI tract that can be seen on a longitudinal image of the left lobe of the liver, just inferior to the heart and anterior to the aorta. This segment is commonly referred to as the
   a. cardiac antrum.
   b. lesser omentum.
   c. esophageal crus.
   d. esophagogastric junction.

7. The visceral layer of the peritoneum lines the walls of the abdominopelvic and the parietal peritioneum covers the organs.
   a. True
   b. False

8. The space between the two layers of peritoneum is known as the peritoneal cavity. It is divided into two parts. Which of the following is one of those parts?
   a. Greater omentum
   b. Mediastinum
   c. Epiploic foramen
   d. Lesser sac

9. An open window opening between the two parts of the peritoneal cavity is called the
   a. greater omentum.
   b. mediastinum.
   c. epiploic foramen.
   d. lesser sac.

10. Which of the structures shown below will not be found within the peritoneum?
    a. Stomach
    b. Pancreas
    c. Cecum
    d. Uterine fundus

19 The Male Pelvis: Prostate Gland and Seminal Vesicles Sonography

I. MEMORIZATION EXERCISE

1. Write the key words in your notebook or on note cards. Write the words on one side of the notepaper and then write the definitions on the opposite side of the page or on the back of the paper. If using note cards, write the key word on the front and the definition on the back. *This step should be completed before the lab session begins.* Memorize the key word definitions silently for 5 minutes, then work with a lab partner and identify the words you still need help with. List the words here. Add additional rows if needed.

II. COMPREHENSION EXERCISE

1. Work with a lab partner to complete this exercise. You will need to write in your notebook. First, change each objective into a question.

   Example: "Describe the location of the prostate gland and seminal vesicles" becomes "Where are the prostate gland and seminal vesicles located?"

2. Next, write a short answer to the question just created.

   Example: "The prostate gland is a doughnut-like gland that lies inferior to the urinary bladder surrounding the proximal urethra. The seminal vesicles are paired glands that lie posterior to the urinary bladder just superior to the prostate."

   Highlight or circle any part of your answers about which you are unsure, and check the answers in your textbook. If you are still unsure of the answers, put a question mark next to the answer(s) for the review session of the lab.

III. APPLICATION OF ANATOMY AND PHYSIOLOGY EXERCISE

Directions to Students: Work on the following with your lab partner.
1. Label the diagram of the male pelvis. Color the structures.

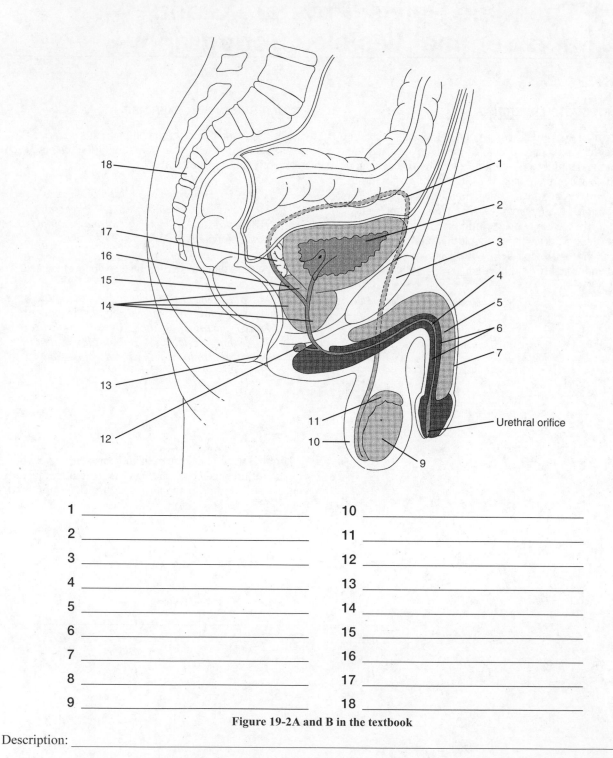

1 _____   10 _____
2 _____   11 _____
3 _____   12 _____
4 _____   13 _____
5 _____   14 _____
6 _____   15 _____
7 _____   16 _____
8 _____   17 _____
9 _____   18 _____

Figure 19-2A and B in the textbook

Description: _____

_____

_____

2. Draw images of the prostate gland and seminal vesicles in longitudinal and transverse planes. Label the zones of the gland. Ask your lab partner to critique your work. What did you miss? Check your drawing using the sketches in your textbook, and complete any missing structures from your drawing. Refer to Figures 19-1 and 19-2 of the textbook to check and correct your answers.

3. Write two or three summary sentences on the physiology of the prostate gland and seminal vesicles. Check your work against the physiology section in the textbook. What else can you add to your description?

_____

_____

_____

IV. IMAGE ANALYSIS EXERCISE

Work on the following figures with a lab partner, a group or independently. The goal is to label correctly all of the sketches and carefully compare the sketch with the sonographic image.

For each sonographic image, write a brief observation that could be "presented" to your instructor, a clinical sonographer, or a sonologist. Please review the section from Chapter 1 on How to Describe Ultrasound Findings. Remember that you want to:

- **recognize** normal echo patterns, so you can identify abnormal presentations,
- **document** differences in echo pattern appearance, and
- **describe** differences in echo pattern appearance using sonographic terminology.

For each image, your assessment should include (1) the view of each major structure (axial or longitudinal) and (2) structures identified in the image with correct sonographic appearance description and measurements if shown.

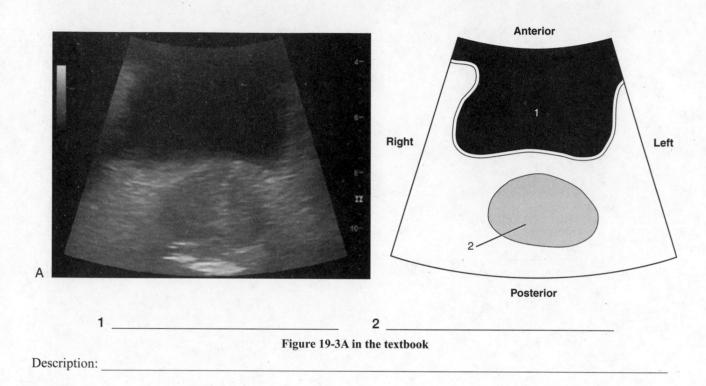

1 _____   2 _____

Figure 19-3A in the textbook

Description: _____
_____
_____

Chapter **19**   **The Male Pelvis: Prostate Gland and Seminal Vesicles Sonography**

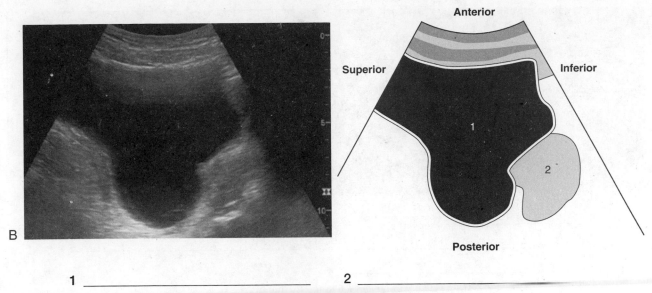

B

1 _____   2 _____

Figure 19-3B in the textbook

Description: _____
_____
_____

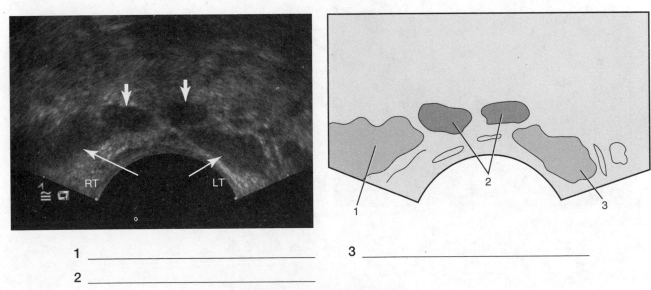

1 _____   3 _____

2 _____

Figure 19-5 in the textbook

Description: _____
_____
_____

Chapter **19**   **The Male Pelvis: Prostate Gland and Seminal Vesicles Sonography**

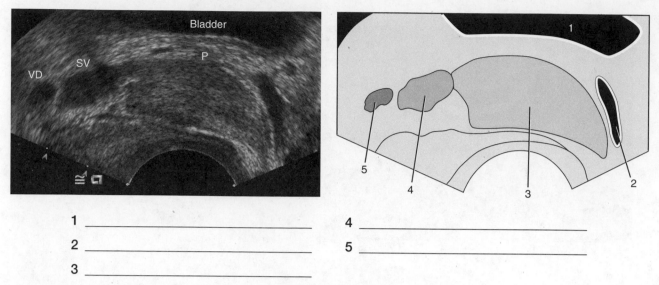

1 _____   4 _____

2 _____   5 _____

3 _____

Figure 19-6 in the textbook

Description: _____

_____

_____

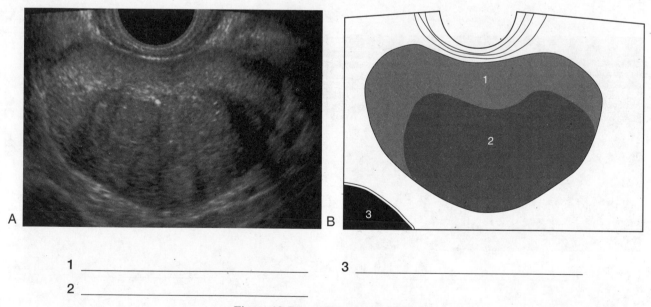

1 _____   3 _____

2 _____

Figure 19-7A and B in the textbook

Description: _____

_____

_____

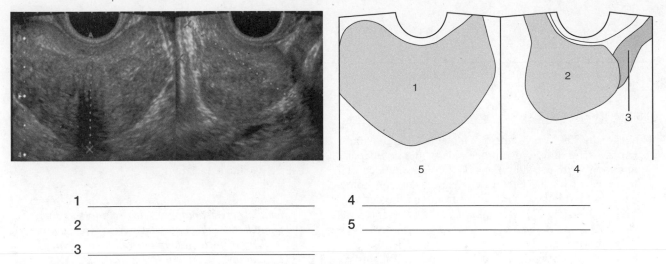

1 _____ 4 _____

2 _____ 5 _____

3 _____

Figure 19-8 in the textbook

Description: _____

_____

_____

V. CHAPTER SUBHEADINGS EXERCISE

1. Convert each chapter subheading into a question; for example, change "Gross Anatomy" to "What is the gross anatomy of the prostate?" Write the answer to each question in a short paragraph in your notebook. Exchange answers with your lab partner and check each other's work. Refer back to the textbook for further information and explanations.

2. What questions do you still have about the chapter? Write your questions in your notebook.

VI. CHAPTER EVALUATION EXERCISE

Use a fresh sheet of notebook paper. Based on your work with the chapter and its accompanying laboratory assignments, identify three concepts you believe are the most important. You may draw from any of the assignments you've already completed in the previous pages including learning objectives, anatomy and physiology, images, or chapter subheadings. Include a detailed rationale in your answers.

Answer the questions below. Refer to page 371 for the answers.

Multiple Choice

1. The length of each seminal vesicle measures approximately
   a. 1 cm.
   b. 5 cm.
   c. 1 mm.
   d. 5 mm.

2. With age, the prostate sometimes
   a. flattens.
   b. calcifies.
   c. enlarges.
   d. atrophies.

3. Of the glandular prostate, the transition zone accounts for about
   a. 5%.
   b. 10%.
   c. 13%.
   d. 33%.

4. Seminal vesicles in the long axis are seen using which scanning plane?
   a. Long.
   b. Axial.
   c. Transverse.
   d. Tangential.

5. The prostate gland is sonographically
   a. asymmetric.
   b. hyperechoic.
   c. homogeneous.
   d. heterogeneous.

True/False

6. The prostate gland and seminal vesicles contribute to sperm viability by secreting alkaline fluids.

7. The fluid secreted by the seminal vesicles constitutes about 33% of semen volume.

8. The seminal vesicles empty into the distal ductus deferens to form the ejaculatory ducts.

9. The transabdominal approach is superior for scanning the seminal vesicles and prostate.

10. The prostate gland consists of a small anterior verumontanum and a much larger posterior glandular region.

I. MEMORIZATION EXERCISE

1. Write the key words in your notebook or on note cards. Write the words on one side of the notepaper and then write the definitions on the opposite side of the page or on the back of the paper. If using note cards, write the key word on the front and the definition on the back. *This step should be completed before the lab session begins.*

   Memorize the key word definitions silently for 5 minutes, then work with a lab partner and identify the words you still need help with. List the words here. Add additional rows if needed.

II. COMPREHENSION EXERCISE

1. Work with a lab partner to complete this exercise. You will need to write in your notebook. First, change each objective into a question.

   Example: "Describe the location of the female pelvic anatomy with relation to the immediate adjacent structures" becomes "Where is the female pelvic anatomy located in relation to adjacent structures?"

2. Next, write a short answer to the question just created.

   Example: "The female pelvis lies in three regions: the right and left iliac, and the hypogastric areas. It is the inferior part of the peritoneal cavity that is bordered by the iliac crests superiorly and the pelvic diaphragm inferiorly."

   Highlight or circle any part of your answers about which you are unsure, and check the answers in your textbook. If you are still unsure of the answers, put a question mark next to the answer(s) for the review session of the lab.

1. Label the diagram of the longitudinal female pelvis as shown in the figure below. Refer to textbook Figure 20-14 to check and correct your answers.

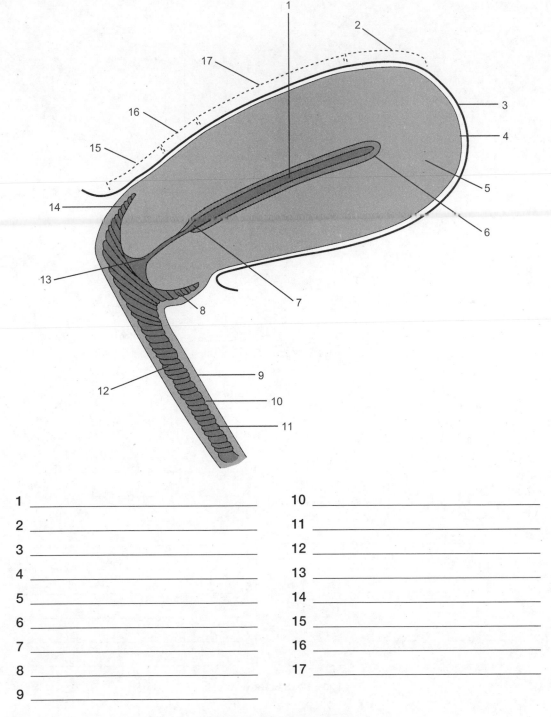

1	_____	10	_____
2	_____	11	_____
3	_____	12	_____
4	_____	13	_____
5	_____	14	_____
6	_____	15	_____
7	_____	16	_____
8	_____	17	_____
9	_____		

Figure 20-14 in the textbook

2. Label the structures of the female pelvis as shown below. Colorize the structures. Refer to Figure 20-15 in the textbook to check and correct your answers.

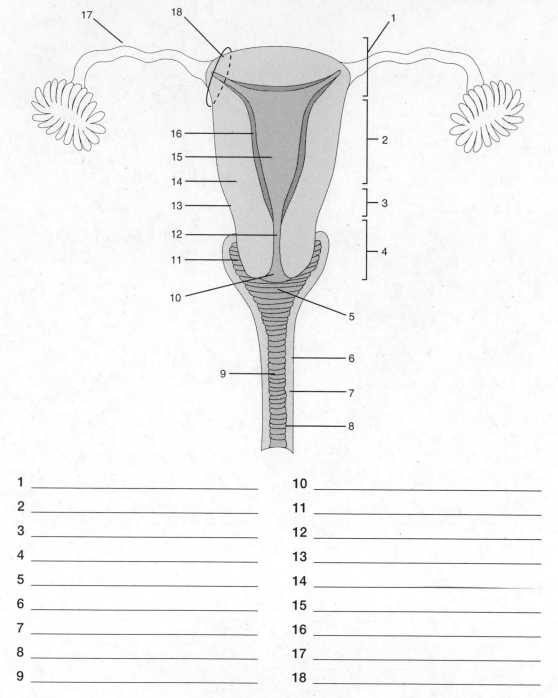

1 _____	10 _____
2 _____	11 _____
3 _____	12 _____
4 _____	13 _____
5 _____	14 _____
6 _____	15 _____
7 _____	16 _____
8 _____	17 _____
9 _____	18 _____

Figure 20-15 in the textbook

3. Label the uterine anomalies in the drawings. Check your answers against textbook Figure 20-12.

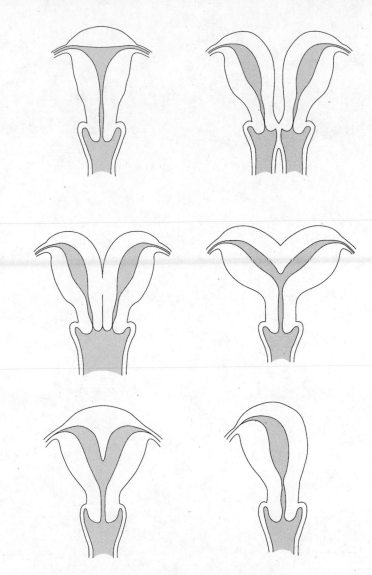

Figure 20-16 in the textbook

4. Label the correct orientation for each of the uterine orientations shown below. Refer to textbook Figure 20-17AD to check your answers.

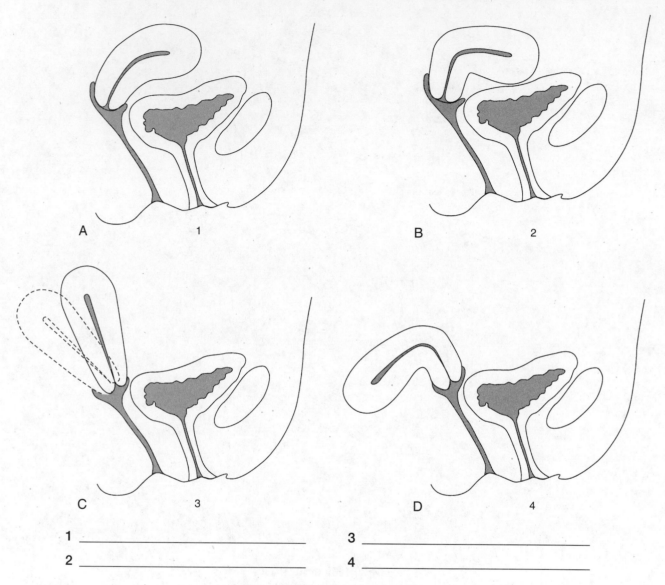

Figure 20-17A to D in the textbook

1 _____   3 _____

2 _____   4 _____

5. Write two or three summary sentences on the physiology of the female pelvis. Ask your lab partner to check your work. Now check your work against the physiology section in the textbook. What else can you add to your description?

_____

_____

_____

_____

_____

IV. IMAGE ANALYSIS EXERCISE

Work on the following figures with a lab partner, a group or independently. The goal is to label correctly all of the sketches and carefully compare the sketch with the sonographic image.

For each sonographic image, write a brief observation that could be "presented" to your instructor, a clinical sonographer, or a sonologist. Please review the section from Chapter 1 on How to Describe Ultrasound Findings. Remember that you want to:

- **recognize** normal echo patterns, so you can identify abnormal presentations,
- **document** differences in echo pattern appearance, and
- **describe** differences in echo pattern appearance using sonographic terminology.

For each image, your assessment should include (1) the view of each major structure (axial or longitudinal) and (2) structures identified in the image with correct sonographic appearance description and measurements if shown.

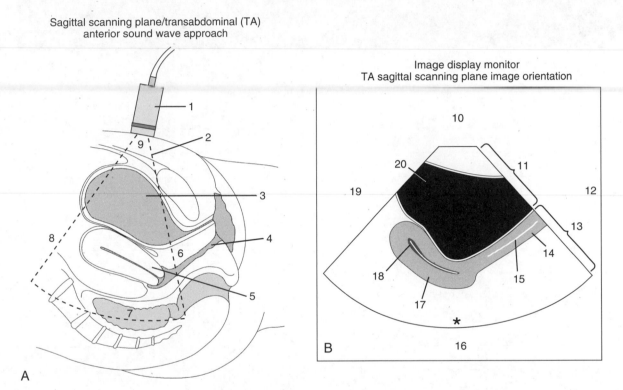

Sagittal scanning plane/transabdominal (TA)
anterior sound wave approach

Image display monitor
TA sagittal scanning plane image orientation

Figure 20-23A and B in the textbook

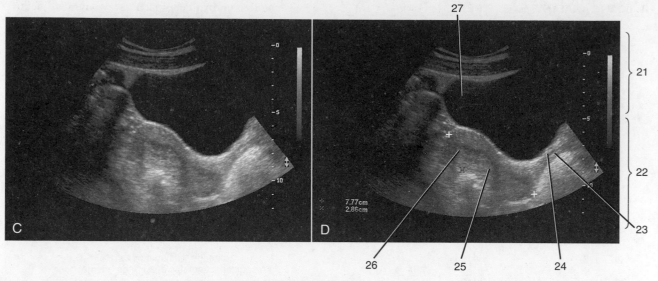

Figure 20-23C and D in the textbook

1 _____
2 _____
3 _____
4 _____
5 _____
6 _____
7 _____
8 _____
9 _____
10 _____
11 _____
12 _____
13 _____
14 _____

15 _____
16 _____
17 _____
18 _____
19 _____
20 _____
21 _____
22 _____
23 _____
24 _____
25 _____
26 _____
27 _____

Figure 20-23C and D in the textbook

Description:

_____
_____
_____

Chapter **20** **The Female Pelvis**

Transverse scanning plane/transabdominal (TA)
anterior sound wave approach

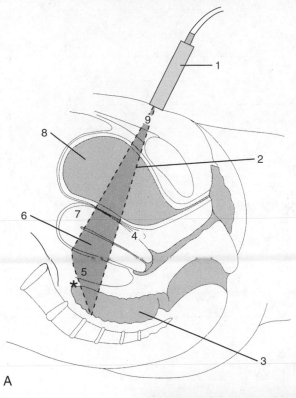

A

Image display monitor
TA transverse scanning plane image orientation

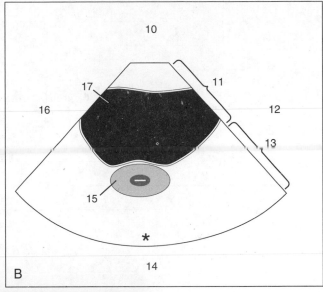

B

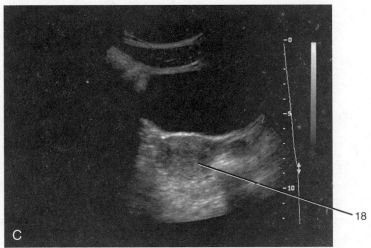

C

1 _____   10 _____
2 _____   11 _____
3 _____   12 _____
4 _____   13 _____
5 _____   14 _____
6 _____   15 _____
7 _____   16 _____
8 _____   17 _____
9 _____   18 _____

Figure 20-24A to C in the textbook

Description:

_____

_____

_____

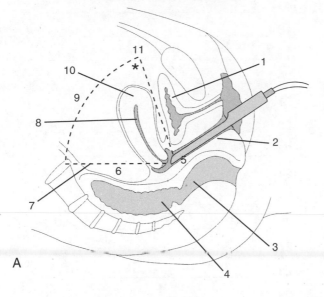

Sagittal scanning plane/transvaginal (TV)
inferior sound wave approach

11
10
9
8
7
6
5
4
3
2
1
*

A

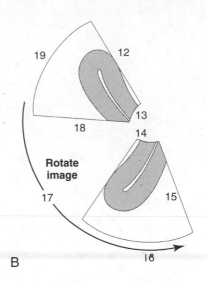

TV sagittal scanning plane image orientation

19
12
13
18
14
15
17
16

**Rotate
image**

B

Image display monitor
TV sagittal scanning plane orientation

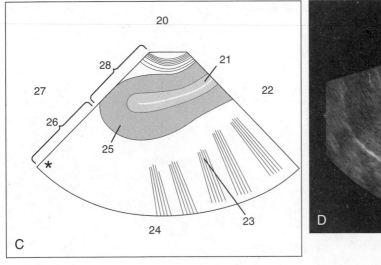

20
21
22
23
24
25
26
27
28
*

C

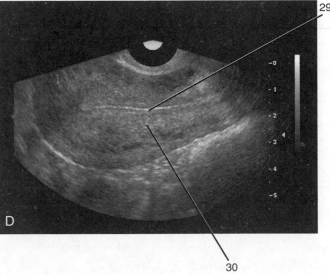

29
30

D

Figure 20-25A to D in the textbook

1 _____

2 _____

3 _____

4 _____

5 _____

6 _____

7 _____

8 _____

9 _____

10 _____

11 _____

12 _____

13 _____

14 _____

15 _____

16 _____

17 _____

18 _____

19 _____

20 _____

21 _____

22 _____

23 _____

24 _____

25 _____

26 _____

27 _____

28 _____

29 _____

30 _____

Figure 20-25A to D in the textbook

Description:

_____

_____

_____

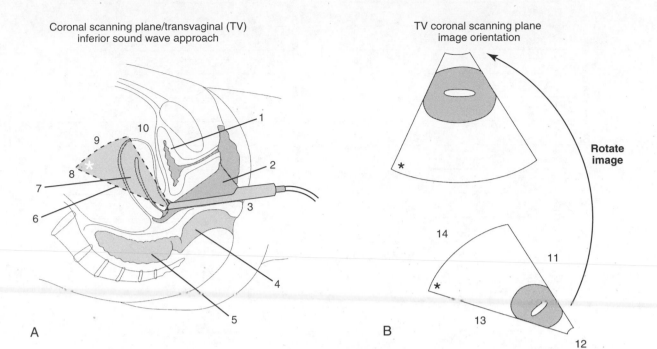

Coronal scanning plane/transvaginal (TV)
inferior sound wave approach

A

TV coronal scanning plane
image orientation

Rotate image

B

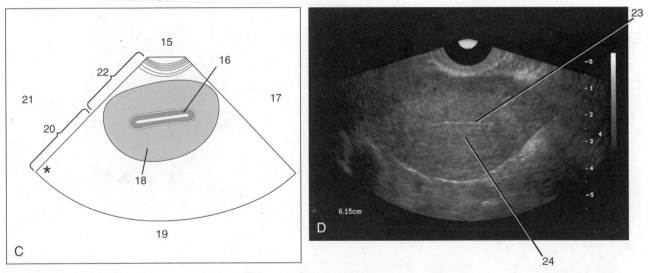

Image display monitor
TV coronal scanning plane orientation

C

D

6.15cm

Figure 20-26A to D in the textbook

1 _____ 13 _____

2 _____ 14 _____

3 _____ 15 _____

4 _____ 16 _____

5 _____ 17 _____

6 _____ 18 _____

7 _____ 19 _____

8 _____ 20 _____

9 _____ 21 _____

10 _____ 22 _____

11 _____ 23 _____

12 _____ 24 _____

Figure 20-26A to D in the textbook

Description:

_____

_____

_____

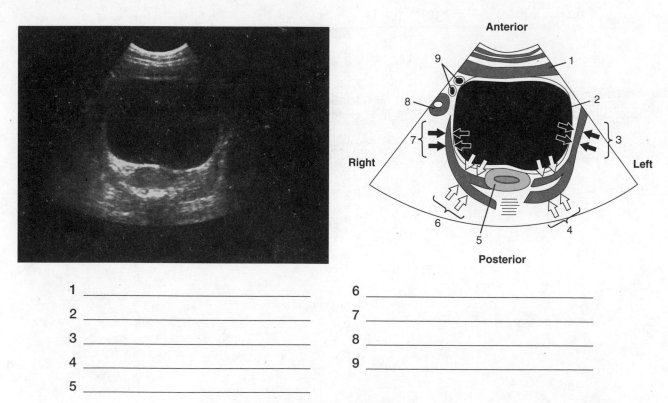

1 _____ 6 _____

2 _____ 7 _____

3 _____ 8 _____

4 _____ 9 _____

5 _____

Figure 20-32 in the textbook

Description:

_____

_____

_____

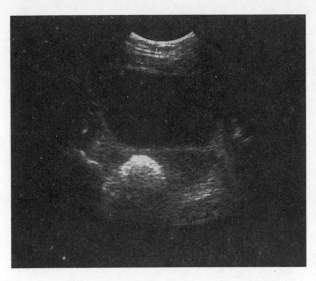
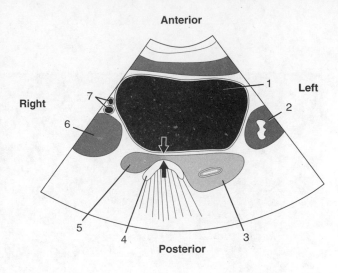

1	_____	5	_____
2	_____	6	_____
3	_____	7	_____
4	_____		

Figure 20-35 in the textbook

Description:

_____

_____

_____

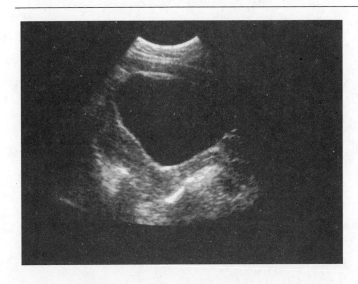

1	_____	4	_____
2	_____	5	_____
3	_____	6	_____

Figure 20-36 in the textbook

Description:

_____

_____

_____

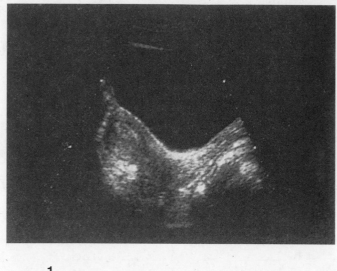

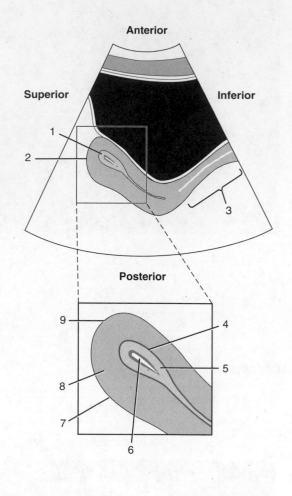

1 _____

2 _____

3 _____

4 _____

5 _____

6 _____

7 _____

8 _____

9 _____

Figure 20-38 in the textbook

Description:

_____

_____

_____

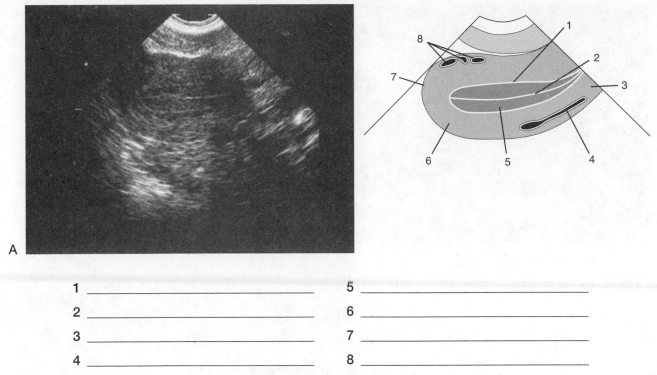

A

1	_____	5	_____
2	_____	6	_____
3	_____	7	_____
4	_____	8	_____

Figure 20-40A in the textbook

Description:

_____

_____

_____

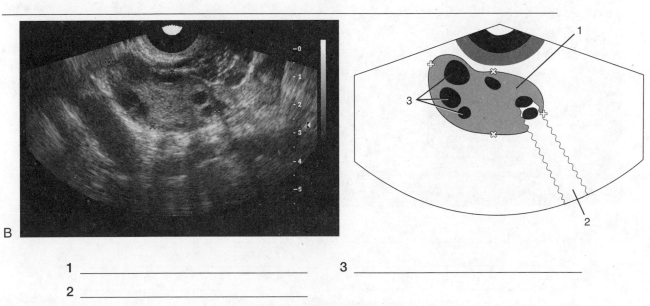

B

1	_____	3	_____
2	_____		

Figure 20-47B in the textbook

Description:

_____

_____

_____

201

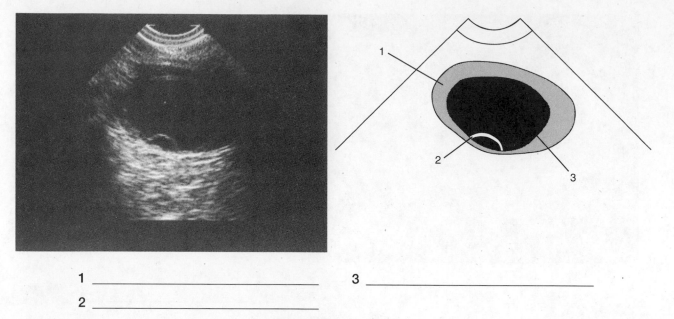

1 _____ 3 _____

2 _____

Figure 20-48 in the textbook

Description:

_____

_____

_____

A

1 _____ 4 _____

2 _____ 5 _____

3 _____ 6 _____

Figure 20-50A in the textbook

Description:

_____

_____

_____

Chapter **20** **The Female Pelvis**

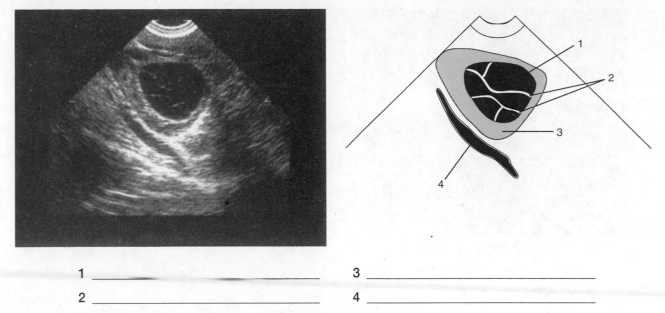

1 _____	3 _____
2 _____	4 _____

Figure 20-51 in the textbook

Description:

_____

_____

_____

A

1 _____	3 _____
2 _____	

Figure 20-57A in the textbook

Description:

_____

_____

_____

Chapter **20**   **The Female Pelvis**

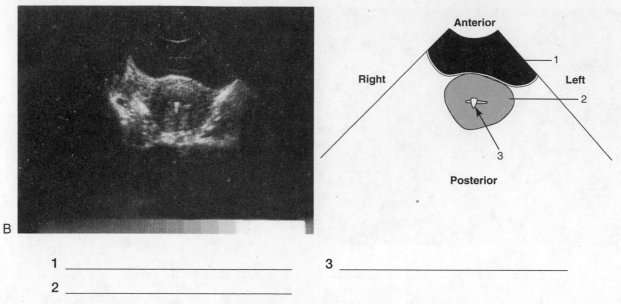

1 _____   3 _____

2 _____

Figure 20-57B in the textbook

Description:

_____

_____

_____

V. CHAPTER SUBHEADINGS EXERCISE

1. Convert each chapter subheading into a question; for example, change "Gross Anatomy" to "What is the gross anatomy of the female pelvis?" Write the answer to each question in a short paragraph in your notebook. Exchange answers with your lab partner and check each other's work. Refer back to the textbook for further information and explanations.
2. What questions do you still have about the chapter? Write your questions in your notebook.

VI. CHAPTER EVALUATION EXERCISE

Use a fresh sheet of notebook paper. Based on your work with the chapter and its accompanying laboratory assignments, identify three concepts you believe are the most important. You may draw from any of the assignments you've already completed in the previous pages including learning objectives, anatomy and physiology, images, or chapter subheadings. Include a detailed rationale in your answers.

Answer the questions below. Refer to page 371 for the answers.

Multiple Choice

1. What is the name of the regions of the true pelvis located posterior to the broad ligaments?
   a. Pelvic cavity
   b. Pelvis major
   c. Adnexa
   d. Pelvic diaphragm

2. _____ are double folds of peritoneum that extend from the uterine cornua to the lateral pelvic walls and provide minor support for the uterus.
   a. Linea terminalis
   b. Spiral bands
   c. Broad ligaments
   d. Circular muscularis

3. Which layer of the uterine wall comprises the bulk of the uterus?
   a. Serosal
   b. Endometrium
   c. Myometrium
   d. Parametrium

4. The palpable external landmark that aids in evaluating the pelvis and is formed from an anterior fusion of bones is known as the
   a. pubic symphysis.
   b. pelvic inlet.
   c. space of Retzius.
   d. ischium.

5. The innominate bones encircle and form the lateral and anterior margins of the
   a. iliac crest.
   b. pelvic diaphragm.
   c. greater sac.
   d. pelvic cavity.

6. Which is not part of the innominate bones?
   a. Ilium
   b. Sacrum
   c. Ischium
   d. Pubis

7. Which false pelvic muscles appear closest to the anterior abdominal wall on transverse sonographic images?
   a. Piriformis
   b. Obturator internus
   c. Iliopsoas
   d. Levator ani

8. Which muscle pairs may be visualized outside the pelvic diaphragm?
   a. Obturator internus
   b. Pubococcygeus
   c. Levator ani
   d. Iliococcygeus

9. Sonographic landmarks of the ovaries include all EXCEPT:
   a. spiral uterine arteries.
   b. external iliac veins.
   c. internal iliac arteries.
   d. iliopsoas muscles.

10. Which of the following sonographic findings are most likely to be visualized when viewing a graafian follicle?
    a. Irregular, thickened walls
    b. Fluid–fluid level
    c. Cellular layers
    d. 20-mm diameter

11. The area imaged in the female pelvis between the uterus and the pubic bone is called the posterior cul de sac. True or False?
    a. True
    b. False

12. The most common of the congenital malformations recognized sonographically by the presence of two endometrial canals that communicate at the level of the cervix is the
    a. uterine didelphys.
    b. bicornuate uterus.
    c. arcuate uterus.
    d. septate uterus.

13. A low resistant Doppler waveform seen in one ovary of the two may help to identify
    a. a dominant follicle.
    b. a postmenopausal woman.
    c. a functional ovary.
    d. a and c

14. True or False? In post-menopausal women, ovarian flow cannot be readily detected.
    a. True
    b. False

First Trimester Obstetrics (0 to 12 Weeks) 21

I. MEMORIZATION EXERCISE

Write the key words in your notebook or on note cards. Write the words on one side of the notepaper and then write the definitions on the opposite side of the page or on the back of the paper. If using note cards, write the key word on the front and the definition on the back. *This step should be completed before the lab session begins.*

Memorize the key word definitions silently for 5 minutes, then work with a lab partner and identify the words you still need help with. List the words here. Add additional rows if needed.

II. COMPREHENSION EXERCISE

1. Work with a lab partner to complete this exercise. You will need to write in your notebook. First, change each objective into a question.

   Example: "Describe the sonographic appearance of the gestational sac and early embryo"

   becomes *"What is the sonographic appearance of the gestational sac and early embryo?"*

2. Next, write a short answer to the question just created.

   Example: "The gestational sac appears on ultrasound as an oval or round, anechoic, fluid-filled sac in the fundus or midportion of the endometrium. A collection of echoes against the wall of the gestational sac represents the early embryo. The gestational sac can be seen as early as 3 weeks' gestational age with transvaginal imaging. The early embryo can be seen at 5 to 6 weeks' gestational age with transvaginal imaging."

Highlight or circle any part of your answers about which you are unsure, and check the answers in your textbook. If you are still unsure of the answers, put a question mark next to the answer(s) for the review session of the lab.

III. APPLICATION OF ANATOMY AND PHYSIOLOGY EXERCISE

1. Label the diagram of normal events in the first four weeks of gestation.

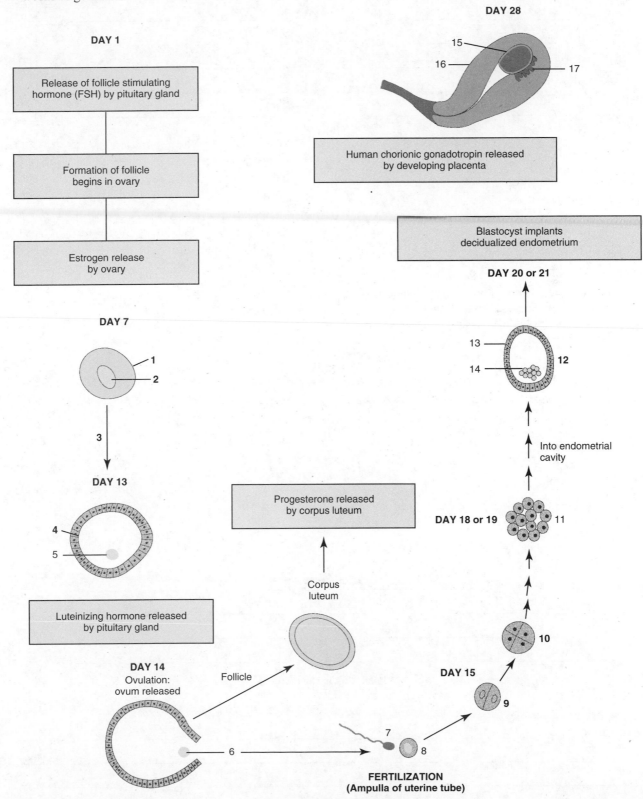

Figure 21-1 in the textbook

1 _____	10 _____
2 _____	11 _____
3 _____	12 _____
4 _____	13 _____
5 _____	14 _____
6 _____	15 _____
7 _____	16 _____
8 _____	17 _____
9 _____	

Figure 21-1 in the textbook

2. Label the diagram of the four to five week gestational sac. Color the structures. Describe the physiology in a few sentences below the diagram.

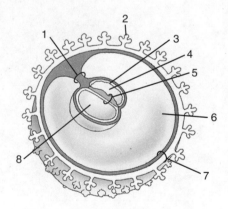

1 _____	5 _____
2 _____	6 _____
3 _____	7 _____
4 _____	8 _____

Figure 21-4 in the textbook

Description: _____

_____

_____

3. Label the diagram of placental development. Color the structures. Describe the physiology in a few sentences below the diagram.

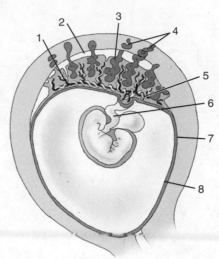

1 _____   5 _____

2 _____   6 _____

3 _____   7 _____

4 _____   8 _____

Figure 21-7 in the textbook

Description: _____

_____

_____

4. Examine the sonogram below. Using the measurements shown, calculate the MSD (mean sac diameter) in centimeters. Compare your answer with that of your lab partners.

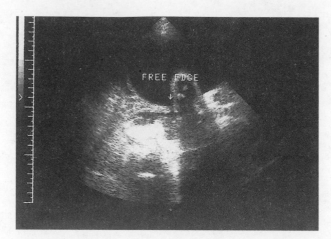

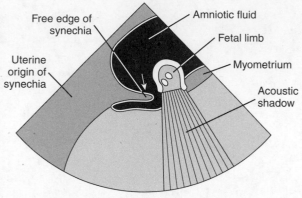

Measurement: _____

Figure 21-25 in the textbook

IV. IMAGE ANALYSIS EXERCISE

Work on the following figures with a lab partner, a group or independently. The goal is to label correctly all of the sketches and carefully compare the sketch with the sonographic image.

For each sonographic image, write a brief observation that could be "presented" to your instructor, a clinical sonographer, or a sonologist. Please review the section from Chapter 1 on How to Describe Ultrasound Findings. Remember that you want to:

- **recognize** normal echo patterns, so you can identify abnormal presentations,
- **document** differences in echo pattern appearance, and
- **describe** differences in echo pattern appearance using sonographic terminology.

For each image, your assessment should include (1) the view of each major structure (axial or longitudinal) and (2) structures identified in the image with correct sonographic appearance description and measurements if shown.

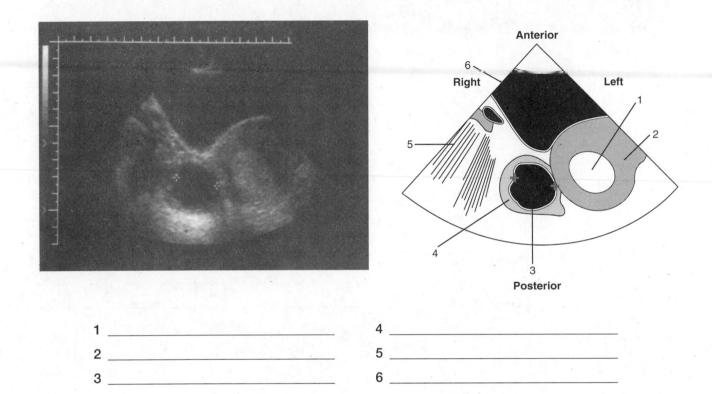

1 _____	4 _____
2 _____	5 _____
3 _____	6 _____

Figure 21-2 in the textbook

Description: _____

_____

_____

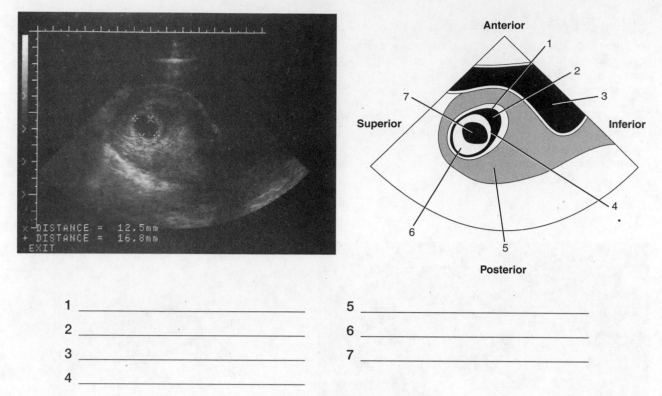

Figure 21-10 in the textbook

1 _____   5 _____

2 _____   6 _____

3 _____   7 _____

4 _____

Description: _____

_____

_____

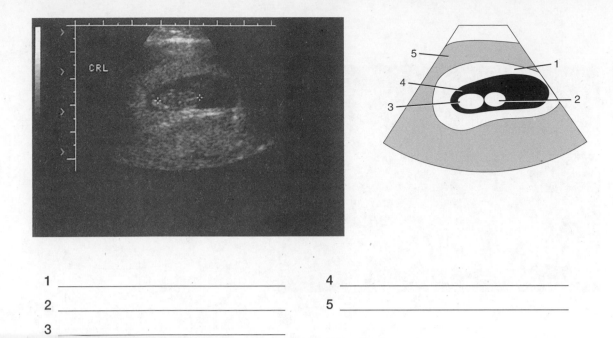

1	_____	4	_____
2	_____	5	_____
3	_____		

Figure 21-13 in the textbook

Description: _____

_____

_____

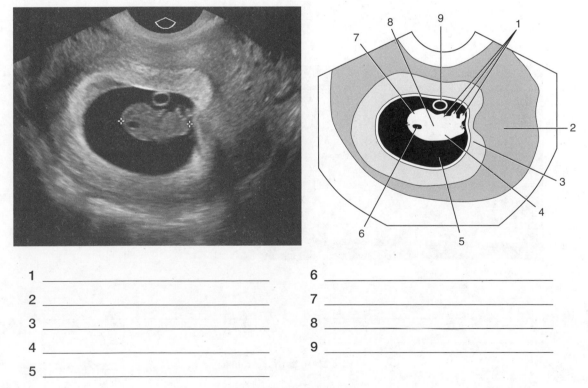

1	_____	6	_____
2	_____	7	_____
3	_____	8	_____
4	_____	9	_____
5	_____		

Figure 21-14 in the textbook

Description: _____

_____

_____

213

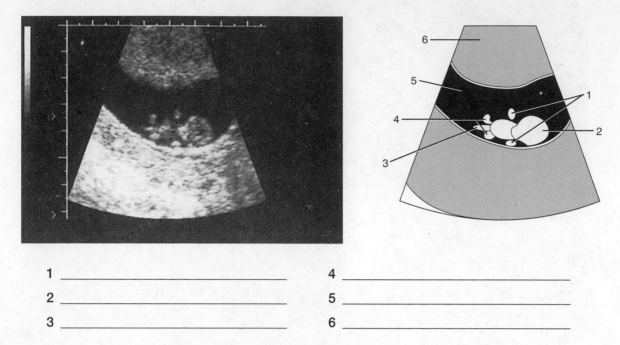

1 _____	4 _____
2 _____	5 _____
3 _____	6 _____

Figure 21-15 in the textbook

Description: _____

_____

_____

1 _____	3 _____
2 _____	

Figure 21-16 in the textbook

Description: _____

_____

_____

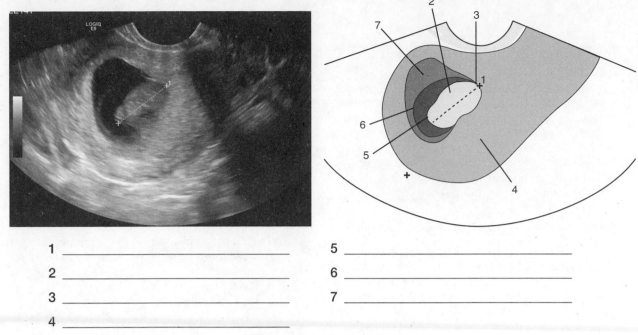

1 _____	5 _____
2 _____	6 _____
3 _____	7 _____
4 _____	

Figure 21-21 in the textbook

Description: _____

_____

_____

1 _____	5 _____
2 _____	6 _____
3 _____	7 _____
4 _____	

Figure 21-24 in the textbook

Description: _____

_____

_____

V. CHAPTER SUBHEADINGS EXERCISE

1. Convert each chapter subheading into a question; for example, change "Development of Fetal Membranes" to "How do the fetal membranes develop?" Write the answer to each question in a short paragraph in your notebook. Exchange answers with your lab partner and check each other's work. Refer back to the textbook for further information and explanations.
2. What questions do you still have about the chapter? Write your questions in your notebook.

VI. CHAPTER EVALUATION EXERCISE

Use a fresh sheet of notebook paper. Based on your work with the chapter and its accompanying laboratory assignments, identify three concepts you believe are the most important. You may draw from any of the assignments you've already completed in the previous pages including learning objectives, anatomy and physiology, images, or chapter subheadings. Include a detailed rationale in your answers.

Answer the questions below. Refer to page 371 for the answers.

Multiple Choice

1. Which of the following terms do sonographers typically use to date a pregnancy?
   a. Conceptual age
   b. Fetal age
   c. Embryonic age
   d. Gestational age

2. Ovulation occurs on the _____ day of the menstrual cycle.
   a. 7th
   b. 14th
   c. 20th
   d. 28th

3. Which hormone causes ovulation, or the release of the egg from the mature follicle?
   a. Estrogen
   b. Progesterone
   c. HCG
   d. Luteinizing hormone

4. The _____ can reach greater than 6 cm in diameter by 7 weeks, and then gradually diminishes.
   a. gestational sac
   b. corpus luteum
   c. amnion
   d. chorion

5. What is the term applied to the functional reaction of the endometrial lining?
   a. Decidua
   b. Amnion
   c. Chorion
   d. Yolk sac

6. The primary yolk sac _____ as the secondary yolk sac forms between the amnion and chorion.
   a. regresses
   b. breaks apart
   c. increases slightly
   d. swells

7. The bilaminar embryonic disk becomes the endoderm, mesoderm, and ectoderm layers during the end of the _____ week.
   a. 2nd
   b. 5th
   c. 8th
   d. 12th

8. The fetal heart starts beating at the beginning of the _____ week.
   a. 2nd
   b. 4th
   c. 6th
   d. 8th

9. At approximately 7 or 8 weeks the yolk stalk fuses with the vitelline duct to become the _____.
   a. placenta
   b. chorion
   c. umbilical cord
   d. neural tube

10. The bowel retracts into the embryo by _____ weeks gestation.
    a. 6
    b. 8
    c. 12
    d. 15

22 Second and Third Trimester Obstetrics (13 to 42 Weeks)

I. MEMORIZATION EXERCISE

1. Write the key words in your notebook or on note cards. Write the words on one side of the notepaper and then write the definitions on the opposite side of the page or on the back of the paper. If using note cards, write the key word on the front and the definition on the back. *This step should be completed before the lab session begins.*

   Memorize the key word definitions silently for 5 minutes, then work with a lab partner and identify the words you still need help with. List the words here. Add additional rows if needed.

II. COMPREHENSION EXERCISE

1. Work with a lab partner to complete this exercise. You will need to write in your notebook. First, change each objective into a question.

   Example: "Describe the sonographic appearance of the placenta and its role in supporting gestation" becomes "What is the sonographic appearance of the placenta, and what is its role in supporting gestation?"

   Next, write a short answer to the question just created.

   Example: "The placenta can be visualized as early as 10 weeks as hyperechoic tissue surrounding a portion of the gestational sac. The purpose of the placenta is to provide a large circulatory surface for exchange of fetal nutrients and waste."

   Highlight or circle any part of your answers about which you are unsure, and check the answers in your textbook. If you are still unsure of the answers, put a question mark next to the answer(s) for the review session of the lab.

III. APPLICATION OF ANATOMY AND PHYSIOLOGY EXERCISE

Work on the following with your lab partner or independently.

1. In your notebook, draw the four grades of the placenta. Color the drawing. Refer to Figure 22.3 in the textbook to check your work.

2. Label as many structures as you can in figures shown of the fetal portal venous circulation and umbilical circulation. Ask your lab partner to critique your work. What did you miss?

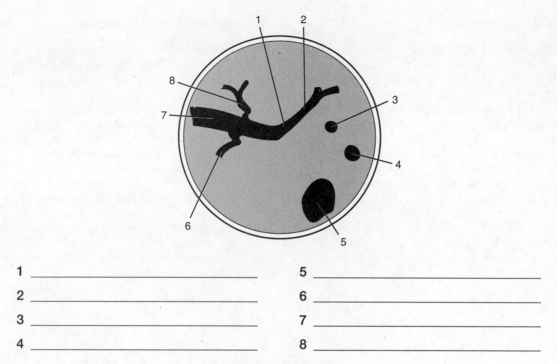

1 _____		5 _____	
2 _____		6 _____	
3 _____		7 _____	
4 _____		8 _____	

Figure 22-13 in the textbook

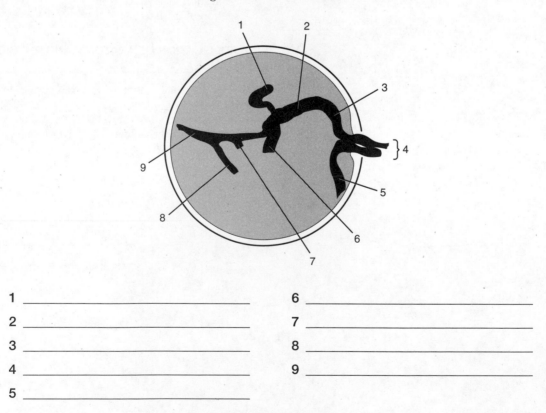

1 _____		6 _____	
2 _____		7 _____	
3 _____		8 _____	
4 _____		9 _____	
5 _____			

Figure 22-14 in the textbook

3. Color and label the fetal heart.

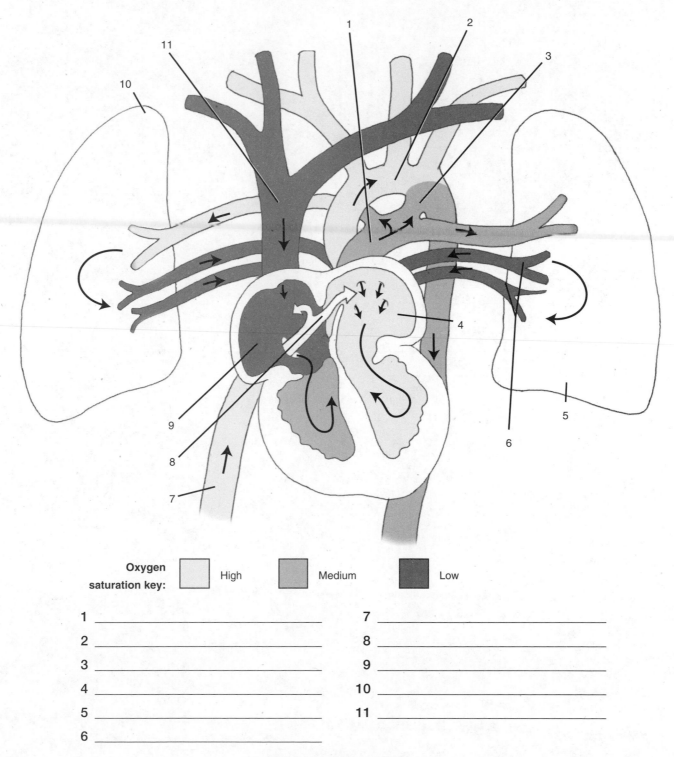

Oxygen saturation key: ▢ High ▢ Medium ▢ Low

1 _____   7 _____
2 _____   8 _____
3 _____   9 _____
4 _____   10 _____
5 _____   11 _____
6 _____

Figure 22-16 in the textbook

Chapter **22** **Second and Third Trimester Obstetrics (13 to 42 Weeks)**

4. Label the structures of the fetal brain at the level of the biparietal diameter.

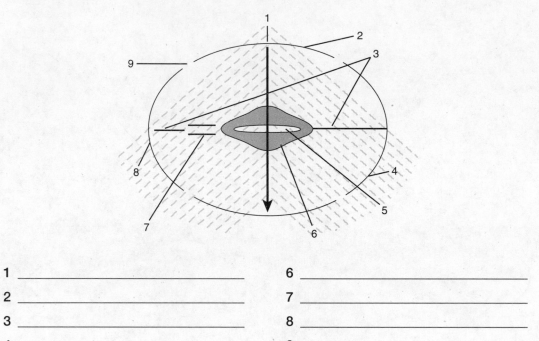

1 _____   6 _____
2 _____   7 _____
3 _____   8 _____
4 _____   9 _____
5 _____

Figure 22-34 in the textbook

IV. IMAGE ANALYSIS EXERCISE

For each sonographic image, write a brief observation that could be "presented" to your instructor, a clinical sonographer, or a sonologist. Please review the section from Chapter 1 on How to Describe Ultrasound Findings. Remember that you want to:

- **recognize** normal echo patterns, so you can identify abnormal presentations,

- **document** differences in echo pattern appearance, and
- **describe** differences in echo pattern appearance using sonographic terminology.

For each image, your assessment should include (1) the view of each major structure (axial or longitudinal) and (2) structures identified in the image with correct sonographic appearance description and measurements if shown.

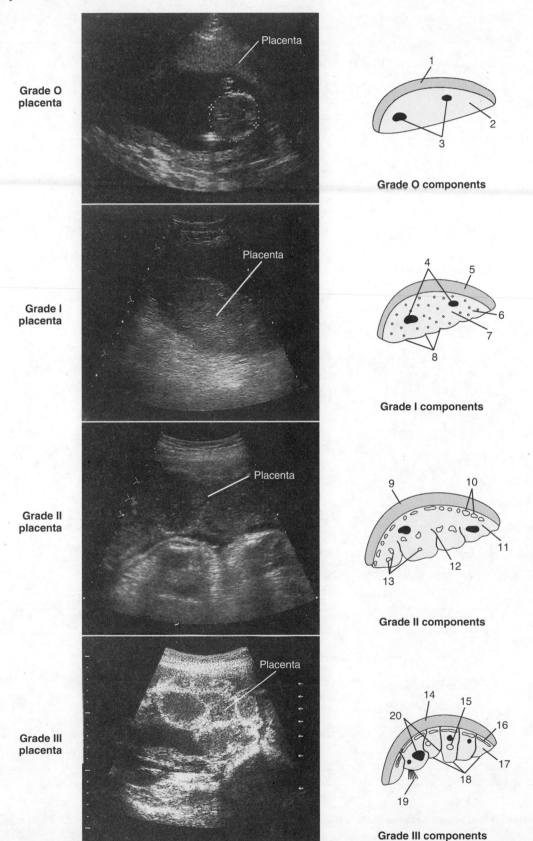

Grade O placenta

Grade I placenta

Grade II placenta

Grade III placenta

Grade O components

Grade I components

Grade II components

Grade III components

1 _____   11 _____
2 _____   12 _____
3 _____   13 _____
4 _____   14 _____
5 _____   15 _____
6 _____   16 _____
7 _____   17 _____
8 _____   18 _____
9 _____   19 _____
10 _____ 20 _____

Figure 22-3 in the textbook

Description:

_____
_____
_____

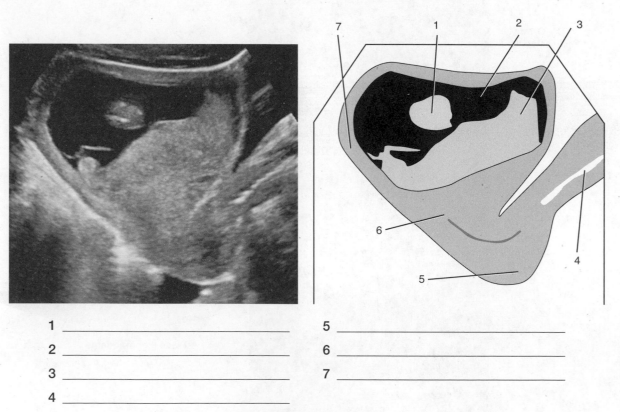

1 _____   5 _____
2 _____   6 _____
3 _____   7 _____
4 _____

Figure 22-4 in the textbook

Description:

_____
_____
_____

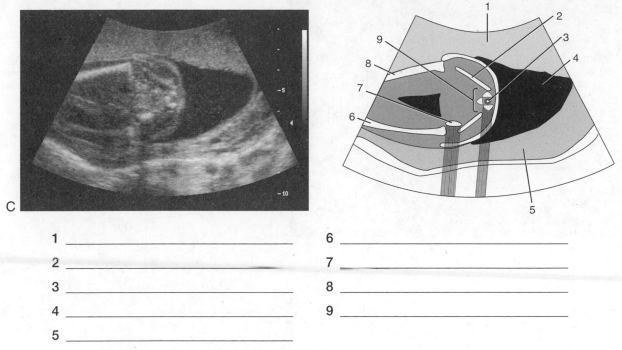

1 _____	6 _____
2 _____	7 _____
3 _____	8 _____
4 _____	9 _____
5 _____	

Figure 22-7C in the textbook

Description:
_____
_____
_____
_____

1 _____	3 _____
2 _____	4 _____

Figure 22-8 in the textbook

Description:
_____
_____
_____

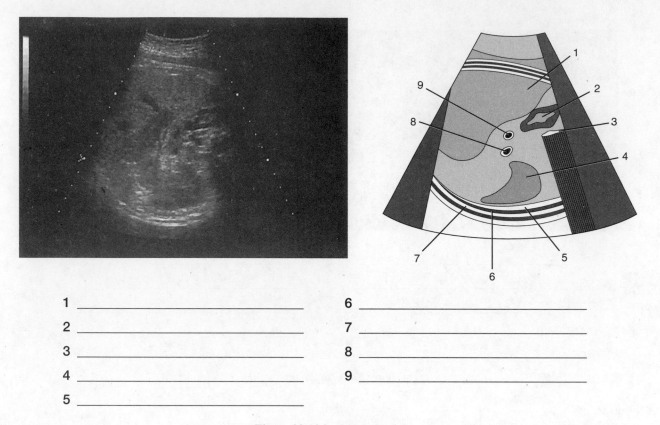

Figure 22-12 in the textbook

1 _____	6 _____
2 _____	7 _____
3 _____	8 _____
4 _____	9 _____
5 _____	

Description:

_____

_____

_____

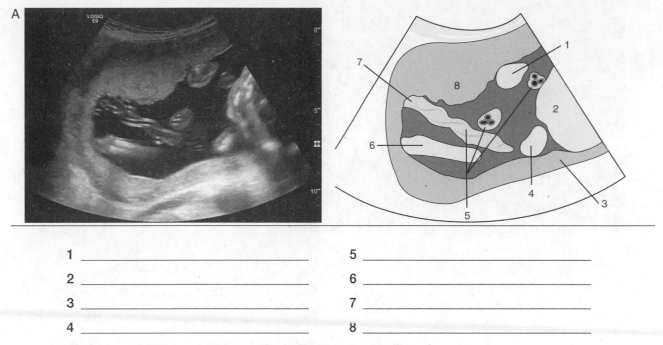

A

1 _____	5 _____
2 _____	6 _____
3 _____	7 _____
4 _____	8 _____

Figure 22-15A in the textbook

(Scan courtesy St. Joseph/Candler Hospital, Ultrasound Department, Savannah, Georgia.)

Description:

_____

_____

_____

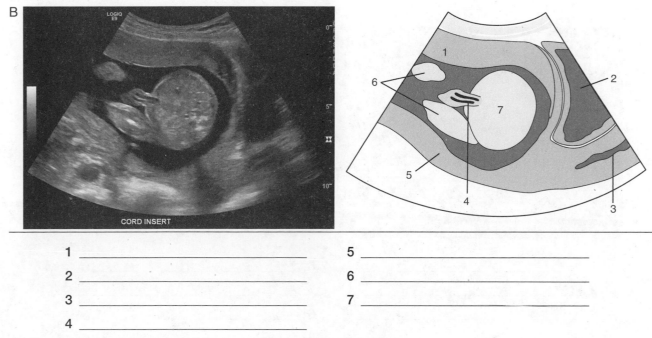

B

1 _____	5 _____
2 _____	6 _____
3 _____	7 _____
4 _____	

Figure 22-15B in the textbook

(Scan courtesy St. Joseph/Candler Hospital, Ultrasound Department, Savannah, Georgia.)

Description:

_____

_____

_____

Chapter **22** **Second and Third Trimester Obstetrics (13 to 42 Weeks)**

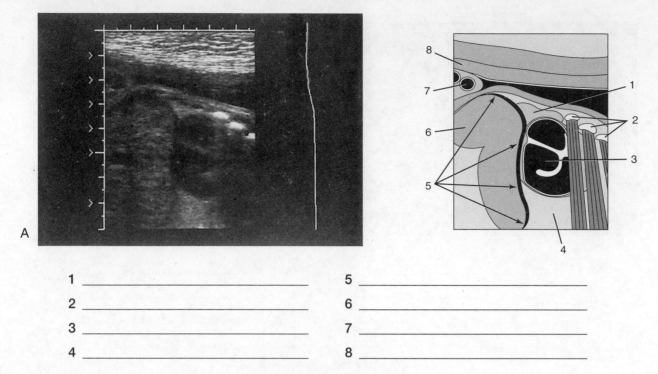

A

1 _____   5 _____

2 _____   6 _____

3 _____   7 _____

4 _____   8 _____

Figure 22-22A in the textbook

Description:

_____

_____

_____

B

1 _____   6 _____

2 _____   7 _____

3 _____   8 _____

4 _____   9 _____

5 _____

Figure 22-22B in the textbook

Description:

_____

_____

_____

Chapter **22** **Second and Third Trimester Obstetrics (13 to 42 Weeks)**

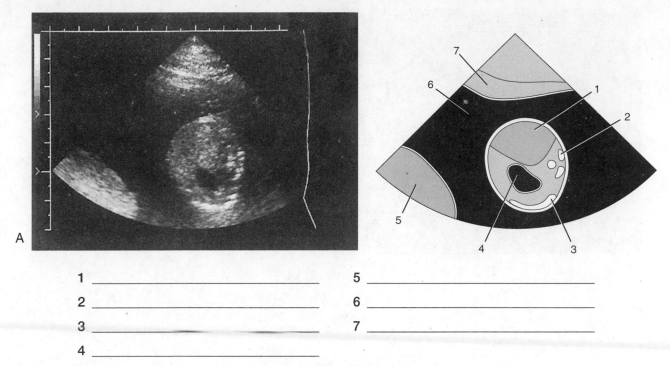

A

1 _____	5 _____
2 _____	6 _____
3 _____	7 _____
4 _____	

Figure 22-23A in the textbook

Description:

_____
_____
_____

B

1 _____	5 _____
2 _____	6 _____
3 _____	7 _____
4 _____	8 _____

Figure 22-23B in the textbook

Description:

_____
_____
_____

Chapter **22   Second and Third Trimester Obstetrics (13 to 42 Weeks)**

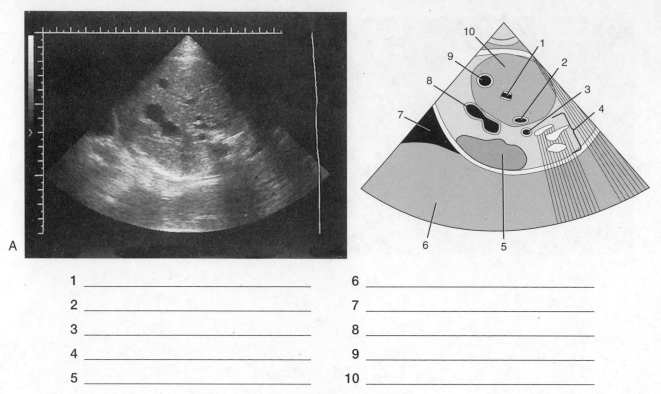

1	_____	6	_____
2	_____	7	_____
3	_____	8	_____
4	_____	9	_____
5	_____	10	_____

Figure 22-24A in the textbook

Description:

_____
_____
_____

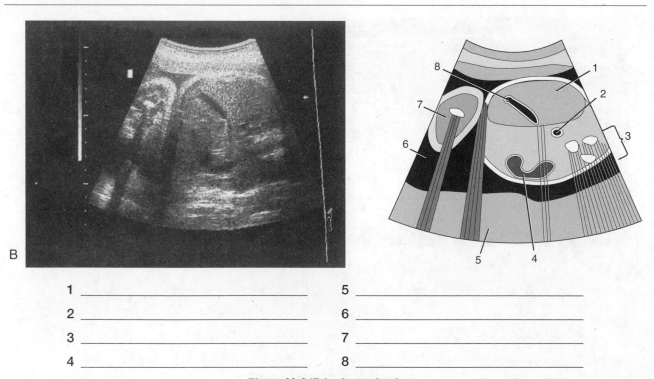

1	_____	5	_____
2	_____	6	_____
3	_____	7	_____
4	_____	8	_____

Figure 22-24B in the textbook

Description:

_____
_____
_____

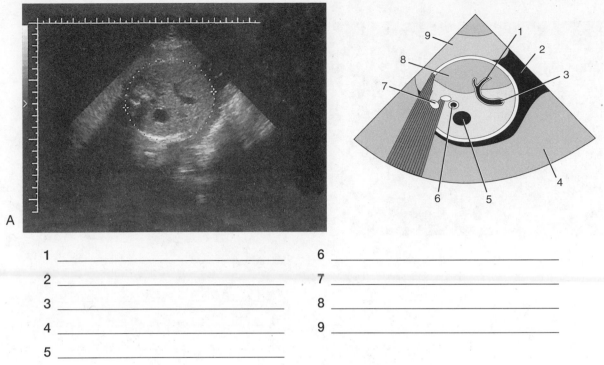

1 _____	6 _____
2 _____	7 _____
3 _____	8 _____
4 _____	9 _____
5 _____	

Figure 22-25A in the textbook

Description:

_____

_____

_____

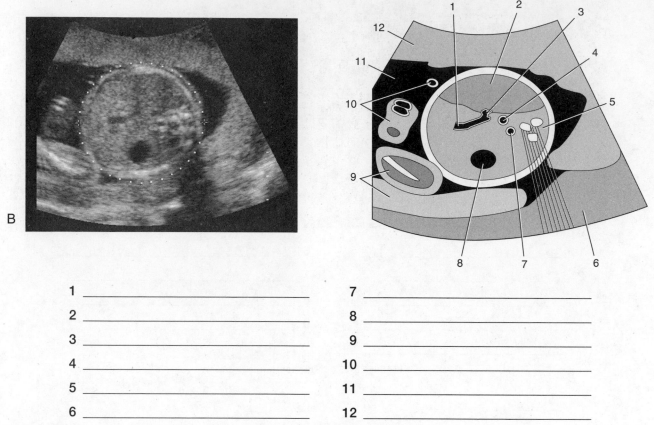

1	_____	7	_____
2	_____	8	_____
3	_____	9	_____
4	_____	10	_____
5	_____	11	_____
6	_____	12	_____

Figure 22-25B in the textbook

(Scan courtesy the University of Virginia Health System, Department of Radiology, Division of Ultrasound, Charlottesville, Virginia.)

Description:

_____

_____

_____

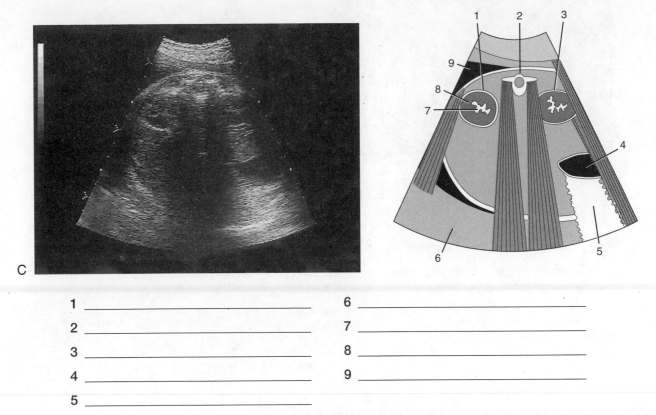

C

1 _____	6 _____
2 _____	7 _____
3 _____	8 _____
4 _____	9 _____
5 _____	

Figure 22-28C in the textbook

Description:

_____

_____

_____

Chapter **22 Second and Third Trimester Obstetrics (13 to 42 Weeks)**

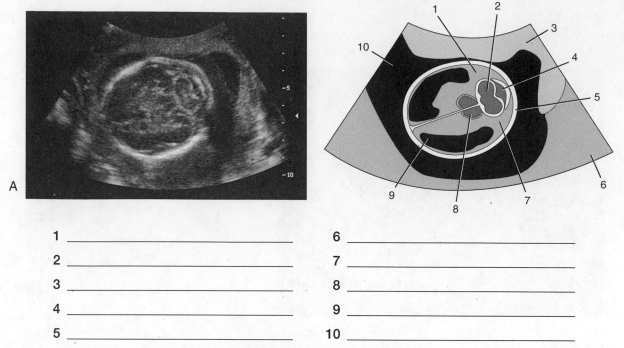

A

1 _____   6 _____
2 _____   7 _____
3 _____   8 _____
4 _____   9 _____
5 _____   10 _____

Figure 22-32A in the textbook

Description:

_____
_____
_____

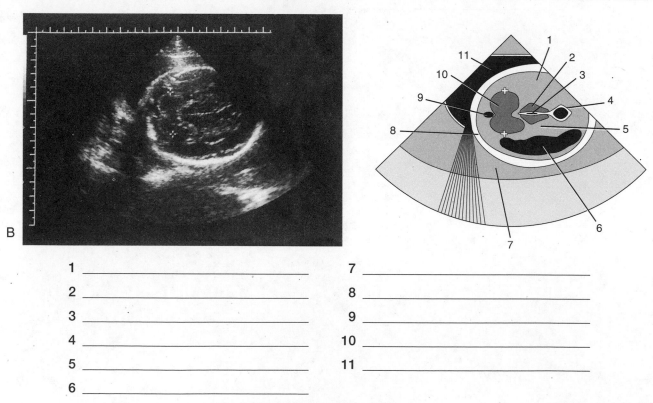

B

1 _____   7 _____
2 _____   8 _____
3 _____   9 _____
4 _____   10 _____
5 _____   11 _____
6 _____

Figure 22-32B in the textbook

Description:

_____
_____
_____

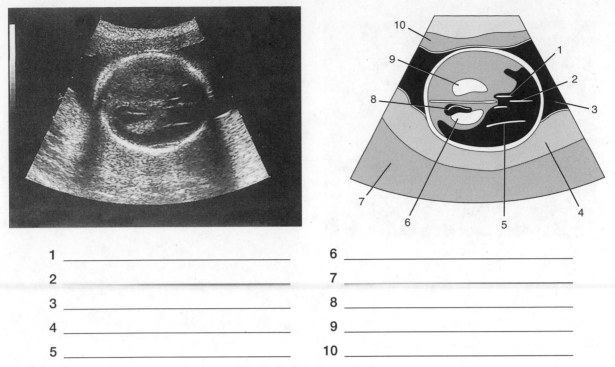

1 _____	6 _____
2 _____	7 _____
3 _____	8 _____
4 _____	9 _____
5 _____	10 _____

Figure 22-33 in the textbook

Description:

_____
_____
_____

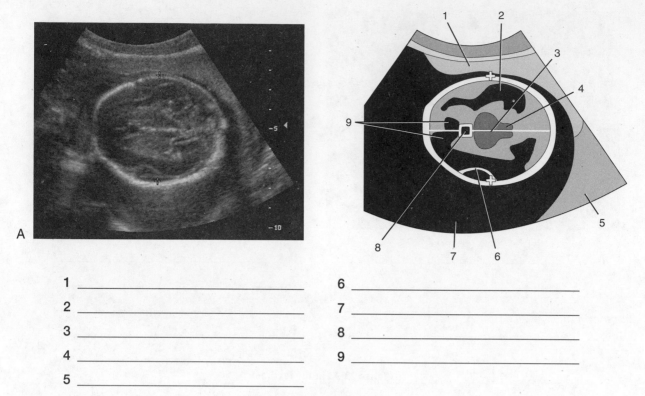

A

1 _____   6 _____

2 _____   7 _____

3 _____   8 _____

4 _____   9 _____

5 _____

Figure 22-35A in the textbook

(Scan courtesy the University of Virginia Health System, Department of Radiology, Division of Ultrasound, Charlottesville, Virginia.)

Description:

_____

_____

_____

V. CHAPTER SUBHEADINGS EXERCISE

1. Convert each chapter subheading into a question; for example, change "The Fetal Organ Systems" to "How do the fetal organs appear on ultrasound?" Write the answer to each question in a short paragraph in your notebook. Exchange answers with your lab partner and check each other's work. Refer back to the textbook for further information and explanations.
2. What questions do you still have about the chapter? Write your questions in your notebook.

VI. CHAPTER EVALUATION EXERCISE

Use a fresh sheet of notebook paper. Based on your work with the chapter and its accompanying laboratory assignments, identify three concepts you believe are the most important. You may draw from any of the assignments you've already completed in the previous pages including learning objectives, anatomy and physiology, images, or chapter subheadings. Include a detailed rationale in your answers.

Answer the questions below. Refer to page 371 for the answers.

Multiple Choice

1. Maternal venous lakes that may interrupt the placenta's homogenous appearance are also called _____.
   a. accreta
   b. previa
   c. lacunae
   d. velamentous

2. _____ is at a much higher concentration in the fetal blood and thus tends to move into the maternal blood.
   a. Oxygen
   b. Carbon dioxide
   c. Nitrogen
   d. Hydrogen

3. In a _____ placenta, the chorionic plate shows some subtle indentation and the homogeneous placental substance exhibits a few scattered, punctate densities that appear hyperechoic relative to the placental substance.
   a. grade 0
   b. grade I
   c. grade II
   d. grade III

4. Normally, a grade II placenta should not appear before _____ weeks.
   a. 36
   b. 37
   c. 38
   d. 39

5. Normal vertebral laminae angle _____.
   a. outward
   b. inward
   c. acutely
   d. obtusely

6. The _____ of the fetal bone attenuates sound waves.
   a. transmission
   b. refraction
   c. density
   d. enhancement

7. Normal fetal muscles appear very _____ on ultrasound.
   a. hyperechoic
   b. echogenic
   c. low-gray
   d. high-gray

8. The umbilical vein connects with the _____ in the fetal liver, transporting oxygenated blood from the placenta to the fetus.
   a. umbilical artery
   b. portal artery
   c. mesenteric vein
   d. portal vein

9. After birth, the _____ eventually becomes the ligamentum teres.
   a. umbilical vein
   b. umbilical artery
   c. falciform ligament
   d. umbilicus

10. What structure of the fetal heart allows blood to move from right to left in the atrial chambers?
    a. Ductus arteriosus
    b. Ductus venosus
    c. Sinus ovale
    d. Foramen ovale

High-Risk Obstetrics 23

I. MEMORIZATION EXERCISE

1. Write the key words in your notebook or on note cards. Write the words on one side of the notepaper and then write the definitions on the opposite side of the page or on the back of the paper. If using note cards, write the key word on the front and the definition on the back. *This step should be completed before the lab session begins.*

   Memorize the key word definitions silently for 5 minutes, then work with a lab partner and identify the words you still need help with. List the words here. Add additional rows if needed.

II. COMPREHENSION EXERCISE

1. Work with a lab partner to complete this exercise. You will need to write in your notebook. First, change each objective into a question.

   Example: "Describe the indications for a biophysical profile" becomes "What are the indications of a biophysical profile?"

   Next, write a short answer to the question just created.

   Example: "The biophysical profile is used to determine fetal well-being. It consists of fetal heart rate, fetal body movements, fetal tone, fetal breathing movements, amniotic fluid volume, and placental grading."

   Highlight or circle any part of your answers about which you are unsure, and check the answers in your textbook. If you are still unsure of the answers, put a question mark next to the answer(s) for the review session of the lab.

III. APPLICATION OF ANATOMY AND PHYSIOLOGY EXERCISE

1. In your notebook, draw the development of monozygotic and dizygotic twins including placentation.

   Label as many structures as you can in each of the drawings. Ask your lab partner to critique your work. What did you miss? Check your drawing using the sketches in your textbook, and complete any missing structures from your drawing.

2. Write two or three summary sentences about the use of ultrasound in high-risk pregnancy. Ask your lab partner to check your work. What else can you add to your description?

IV. IMAGE ANALYSIS EXERCISE

Work on the following figures with your lab partner. It's your choice! You can label all the sketches at once, then go back and label each image with your lab partner, or label an image and its accompanying sketch at the same time. Either way, the goal is to label all of the sketches correctly and carefully compare the sketch with the sonographic image.

For each sonographic image, write a very brief observation that could be presented to your instructor, the clinical sonographer, or the sonologist. Your observation will be based on Chapter 1 in the textbook, which describes how to write a technical observation. Please go back and review that chapter if needed.

For each image, your assessment should include (1) the view of each major structure (axial or longitudinal; note: these are not the scanning planes) and (2) structures identified in the image with the correct sonographic appearance, description, and measurements if shown (see Chapter 1 in the textbook for information on how to write a technical observation).

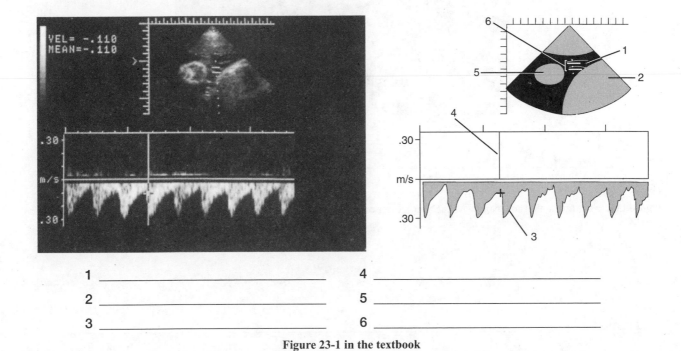

1 _____	4 _____
2 _____	5 _____
3 _____	6 _____

Figure 23-1 in the textbook

Description: _____
_____
_____

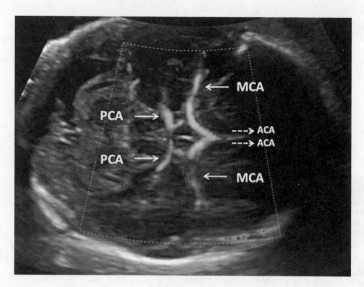

1 _____   4 _____

2 _____   5 _____

3 _____   6 _____

Figure 23-2 in the textbook (From Norton M.E. Callen's Ultrasonography in Obstetrics and Gynecology, 6th ed, Philadelphia, 2017, Elsevier.)

Description: _____

_____

_____

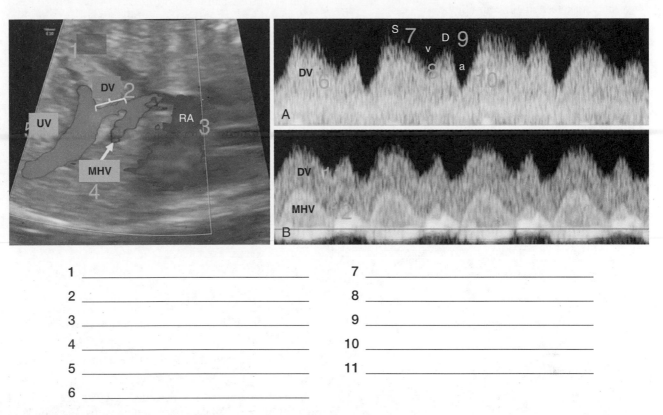

1	_____	7	_____
2	_____	8	_____
3	_____	9	_____
4	_____	10	_____
5	_____	11	_____
6	_____		

Figure 23-3 in the textbook (From Copel J.A., D'Alton M.E., et. al. Obstetric Imaging: Fetal Diagnosis and Care, 2nd ed, Philadelphia, 2018, Elsevier.)

Description: _____

_____

_____

V. CHAPTER SUBHEADINGS EXERCISE

1. Convert each chapter subheading into a question; for example, change "Sonographic Appearance of Multifetal Gestation" to "What is the sonographic appearance of multifetal gestation?" Write the answer to each question in a short paragraph in your notebook. Exchange answers with your lab partner and check each other's work. Refer back to the textbook for further information and explanations.
2. What questions do you still have about the chapter? Write your questions in your notebook.

VI. CHAPTER EVALUATION EXERCISE

Based on your work with the chapter and its accompanying laboratory assignments, identify three concepts you believe are the most important. You may draw from any of the assignments you've already completed in the previous pages including learning objectives, anatomy and physiology, images, or chapter subheadings. Include a detailed rationale in your answers.

1 _____

_____

_____

_____

_____

2 _____

_____

_____

_____

_____

3 _____

_____

_____

_____

_____

Answer the questions below. Refer to page 371 for the answers.

Multiple Choice

1. When performing Doppler studies of placental and fetal circulation, which of the following is best at predicting poor fetal outcome?
   a. Systolic flow
   b. Diastolic flow
   c. High resistant waveform
   d. Low resistant waveform
2. Venous pulsations in the umbilical vein are a normal occurrence up until how many weeks of gestation?
   a. 15 weeks
   b. 18 weeks
   c. 21 weeks
   d. 24 weeks
3. Abnormal ductus venosus velocity is useful in determining all of the following EXCEPT:
   a. Fetal cardiac disease
   b. Severe growth restriction
   c. Fetal congestive heart failure
   d. Fetal anemia
4. To decrease the risk for possible complications, an amniocentesis is ideally performed no earlier than
   a. 14 weeks.
   b. 16 weeks.
   c. 18 weeks.
   d. 20 weeks.

Completion

Assign a score of 0 or 2 for the following scenarios seen in a 30-minute time frame while performing a biophysical profile.

5. The fetus arched its back twice and had one episode of movement of all arms and legs. Score ____

6. The fetus had three episodes of heart accelerations of at least 22 beats per minute lasting 17 seconds in duration, then 15 seconds, then 20 seconds. Score ____

7. The sonographer visualized two episodes of fetal breathing movements, the first lasting 30 seconds and the second lasting 25 seconds. Score ____

8. There was one pocket of amniotic fluid measuring 2.5 cm in vertical diameter that was free of umbilical cord and fetal extremities. Score ____

9. The fetus had his legs bent at the beginning of the exam and the sonographer observed him extend them straight and remain like that during the rest of the exam. Score ____

10. The fetus was observed opening and closing his hand. Score ____

I. MEMORIZATION EXERCISE

1. Write the key words in your notebook or on note cards. Write the words on one side of the notepaper and then write the definitions on the opposite side of the page or on the back of the paper. If using note cards, write the key word on the front and the definition on the back. *This step should be completed before the lab session begins.*

   Memorize the key word definitions silently for 5 minutes, then work with a lab partner and identify the words you still need help with. List the words here. Add additional rows if needed.

II. COMPREHENSION EXERCISE

1. Work with a lab partner to complete this exercise. You will need to write in your notebook. First, change each objective into a question.

   Example: "Describe the location and size of the heart in the fetus" becomes "What is the location and size of the heart in the fetus?"

Next, write a short answer to the question just created.

Example: "The fetal heart is located in the anterior half of the chest with the base of the heart, the atria, in the middle of the chest. The apex of the heart, the tip of the ventricles, is to the left of the midline. The fetal heart is about the size of a quarter at 20 weeks' gestational age."

Highlight or circle any part of your answers about which you are unsure, and check the answers in your textbook. If you are still unsure of the answers, put a question mark next to the answer(s) for the review session of the lab.

III. APPLICATION OF ANATOMY AND PHYSIOLOGY EXERCISE

1. Label the diagram of the blood flow in the fetal heart.

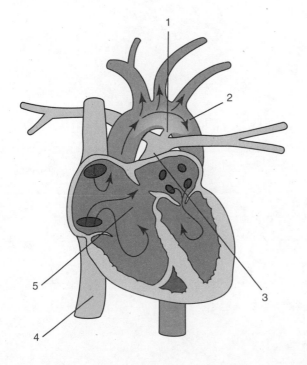

1 _____

2 _____

3 _____

4 _____

5 _____

Figure 24-1 in the text.

2. Label the diagram of fetal circulation.

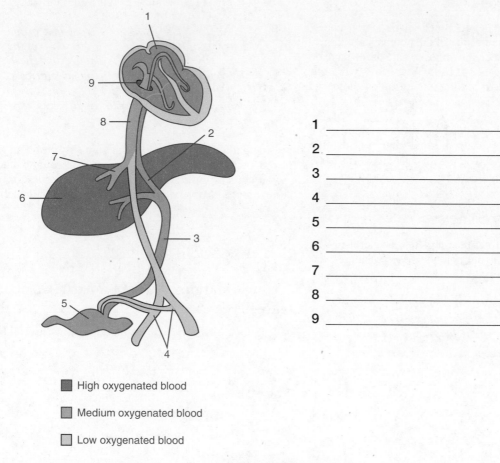

High oxygenated blood

Medium oxygenated blood

Low oxygenated blood

1 _____
2 _____
3 _____
4 _____
5 _____
6 _____
7 _____
8 _____
9 _____

Figure 24-4 in the text

3. Write two or three summary sentences about the physiology of the fetal heart. Ask your lab partner to check your work. Now check your work against the physiology section in the textbook. What else can you add to your description?

_____

_____

_____

_____

_____

IV. IMAGE ANALYSIS EXERCISE

Work on the following figures with a lab partner, a group or independently. The goal is to label correctly all of the sketches and carefully compare the sketch with the sonographic image.

For each sonographic image, write a brief observation that could be "presented" to your instructor, a clinical sonographer, or a sonologist. Please review the section from Chapter 1 on How to Describe Ultrasound Findings. Remember that you want to:

- **recognize** normal echo patterns, so you can identify abnormal presentations,
- **document** differences in echo pattern appearance, and
- **describe** differences in echo pattern appearance using sonographic terminology.

For each image, your assessment should include (1) the view of each major structure (axial or longitudinal) and (2) structures identified in the image with correct sonographic appearance description and measurements if shown.

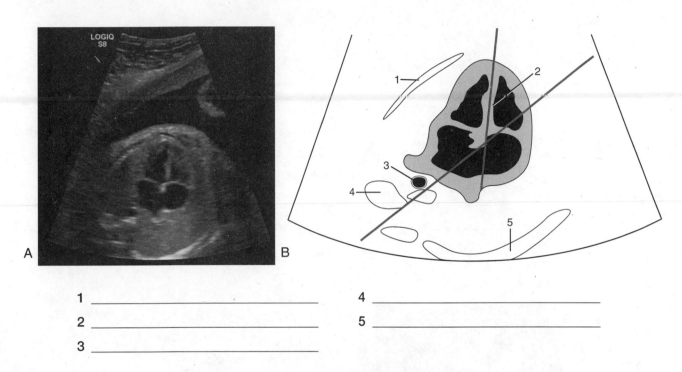

1 _____   4 _____

2 _____   5 _____

3 _____

Figure 24-6 in the text

Description: _____

_____

_____

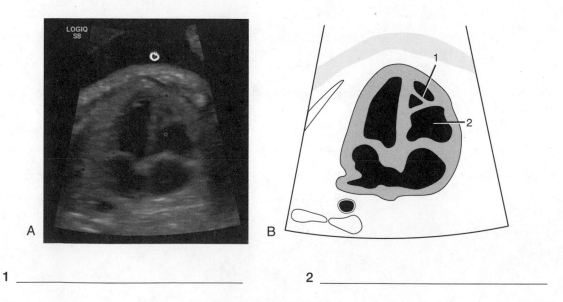

1 _____ 7 _____

2 _____ 8 _____

3 _____ 9 _____

4 _____ 10 _____

5 _____ 11 _____

6 _____ 12 _____

Figure 24-10 in the text

Description: _____

_____

_____

1 _____ 2 _____

Figure 24-11 in the text

Description: _____

_____

_____

Chapter **24 Fetal Echocardiography**

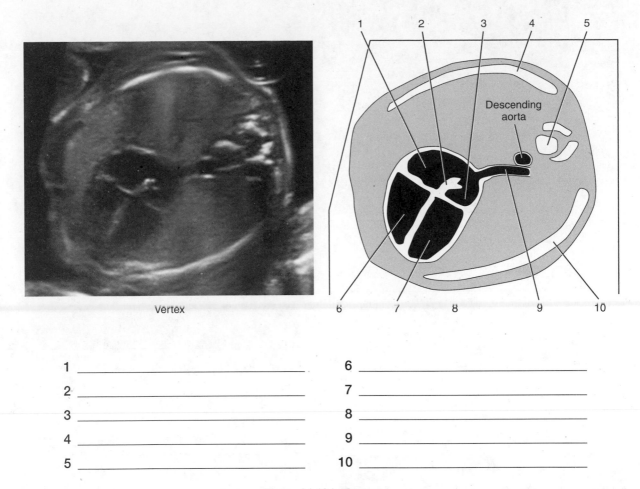

Vertex

1 _____	6 _____
2 _____	7 _____
3 _____	8 _____
4 _____	9 _____
5 _____	10 _____

Figure 24-12 in the text

Description: _____

_____

_____

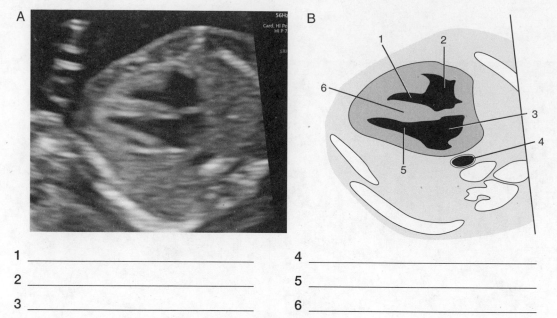

A   B

1 _____   4 _____

2 _____   5 _____

3 _____   6 _____

Figure 24-13 in the text

Description: _____

_____

_____

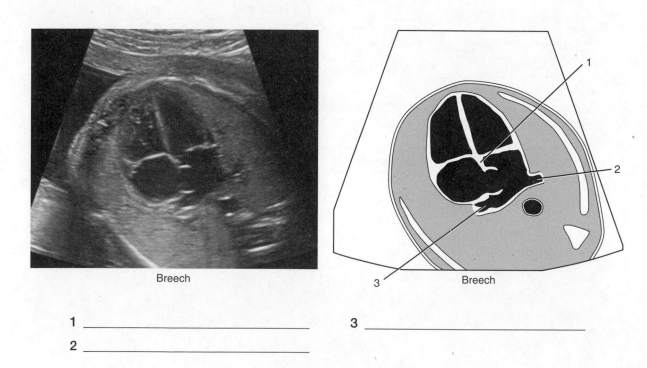

Breech   Breech

1 _____   3 _____

2 _____

Figure 24-14 in the text

Description: _____

_____

_____

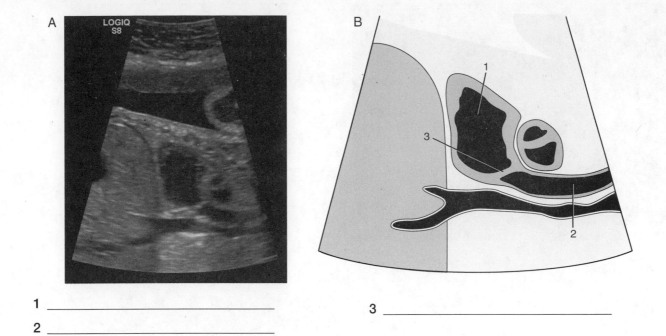

1 _____

2 _____

3 _____

Figure 24-16 in the text

Description: _____

_____

_____

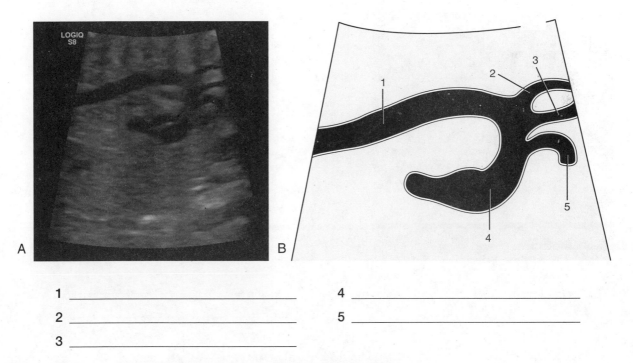

1 _____   4 _____

2 _____   5 _____

3 _____

Figure 24-18 in the text

Description: _____

_____

_____

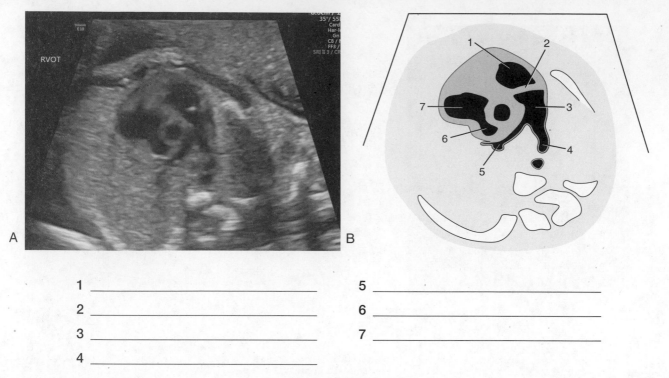

1	_____	5	_____
2	_____	6	_____
3	_____	7	_____
4	_____		

Figure 24-19 in the text

Description: _____

_____

_____

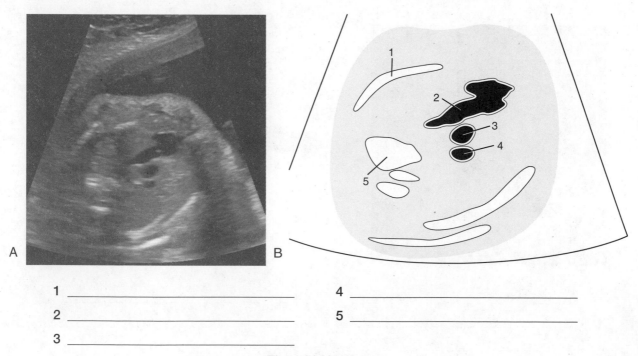

1	_____	4	_____
2	_____	5	_____
3	_____		

Figure 24-23 in the text

Description: _____

_____

_____

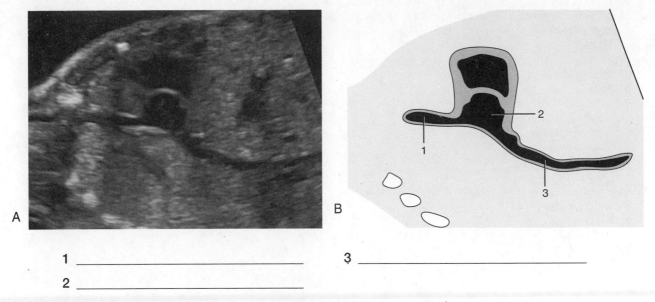

1 _____

2 _____

3 _____

Figure 24-27 in the text

Description: _____

_____

_____

V. CHAPTER SUBHEADINGS EXERCISE

1. Convert each chapter subheading into a question; for example, change "Normal Variants" to "What are the normal variants of the fetal heart?" Write the answer to each question in a short paragraph in your notebook. Exchange answers with your lab partner and check each other's work. Refer back to the textbook for further information and explanations.
2. What questions do you still have about the chapter? Write your questions in your notebook.

VI. CHAPTER EVALUATION EXERCISE

Use a fresh sheet of notebook paper. Based on your work with the chapter and its accompanying laboratory assignments, identify three concepts you believe are the most important. You may draw from any of the assignments you've already completed in the previous pages including learning objectives, anatomy and physiology, images, or chapter subheadings. Include a detailed rationale in your answers.

Answer the questions below. Refer to page 372 for the answers.

Multiple Choice

1. What fetal heart structure allows for blood to flow from the right atrium to the left atrium?
   a. Ductus arteriosus
   b. Foramen ovale
   c. Ductus venosus
   d. Atrial valve
2. What structure aids in distinguishing the right ventricle from the left ventricle in a four-chamber view?
   a. Moderator band
   b. Mitral valve
   c. Pulmonary artery
   d. Pulmonary veins
3. What is the normal axis of the fetal heart within the fetal thorax?
   a. 15 degrees
   b. 30 degrees
   c. 45 degrees
   d. 60 degrees
4. Which valve has an association with the inferior vena cava?
   a. Pulmonary valve
   b. Eustachian valve
   c. Aortic valve
   d. Tricuspid valve
5. How is oxygenated blood provided to the fetus?
   a. Umbilical vein
   b. Umbilical artery
   c. Fetal lungs
   d. Pulmonary veins

6. What is the approximate size of the fetal heart at 20 weeks' gestation?
    a. 20 mm
    b. 25 mm
    c. 30 mm
    d. 35 mm
7. Which fetal shunt provides blood flow directly to the descending aorta?
    a. Foramen ovale
    b. Ductus venosus
    c. Atrial valve
    d. Ductus arteriosus
8. In a four-chamber view, what structure lies closest to the anterior chest wall?
    a. Right atrium
    b. Left atrium
    c. Right ventricle
    d. Left ventricle
9. Which view is best for visualizing muscular intra-ventricular septum defects?
    a. Subcostal four-chamber view
    b. LVOT
    c. Bicaval view
    d. RVOT
10. How many pulmonary veins are typically connected to the left atrium?
    a. 2
    b. 3
    c. 4
    d. 5

25 The Neonatal Brain

I. MEMORIZATION EXERCISE

1. Write the key words in your notebook or on note cards. Write the words on one side of the notepaper and then write the definitions on the opposite side of the page or on the back of the paper. If using note cards, write the key word on the front and the definition on the back. *This step should be completed before the lab session begins.*

    Memorize the key word definitions silently for 5 minutes, then work with a lab partner and identify the words you still need help with. List the words here. Add additional rows if needed.

II. COMPREHENSION EXERCISE

1. Work with a lab partner to complete this exercise. You will need to write in your notebook. First, change each objective into a question.

    Example: "Identify the major structures in the neonatal brain" becomes "What are the major structures in the neonatal brain?"

    Next, write a short answer to the question just created.

    Example: "The brain has four major regions: cerebral hemispheres, diencephalon, brain stem, and cerebellum. The cerebral hemispheres are further divided into frontal, parietal, temporal, and occipital lobes. The diencephalon, also called the interbrain, rests superior to the brain stem, is enclosed by the cerebral hemispheres, and comprises the thalamus, hypothalamus, and epithalamus. The brain stem comprises the midbrain, pons, and medulla oblongata. The cerebellum is located anterior to the brain stem."

Highlight or circle any part of your answers about which you are unsure, and check the answers in your textbook. If you are still unsure of the answers, put a question mark next to the answer(s) for the review session of the lab.

III. APPLICATION OF ANATOMY AND PHYSIOLOGY EXERCISE

Work on the following with your lab partner.

1. In your notebook, draw the brain lobes from memory. Label the brain and lobes; include each structure's orientation in the body (either vertical, horizontal, vertical oblique, or horizontal oblique). Ask your lab partner to critique your work. What did you miss?

2. Write two or three summary sentences about the physiology of the neonatal brain. Ask your lab partner to check your work. Now check your work against the physiology section in the textbook. What else can you add to your description?

IV. IMAGE ANALYSIS EXERCISE

Work on the following figures with your lab partner. It's your choice! You can label all the sketches at once, then go back and label each image with your lab partner, or label an image and its accompanying sketch at the same time. Either way, the goal is to label correctly all of the sketches and carefully compare the sketch with the sonographic image.

For each sonographic image, write a brief observation that could be "presented" to your instructor, a clinical sonographer, or a sonologist. Please review the section from Chapter 1 on How to Describe Ultrasound Findings. Remember that you want to:

- **differentiate** abnormal echo patterns from normal echo patterns,
- **document** any differences in echo pattern appearance, and
- **describe** any difference in echo pattern appearance using sonographic terminology.

For each image, your assessment should include (1) the view of each major structure (axial or longitudinal; note: these are not the scanning planes) and (2) structures identified in the image with correct sonographic appearance description and measurements if shown.

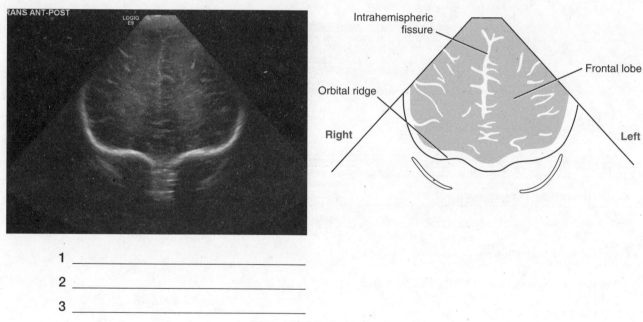

1 _____

2 _____

3 _____

Figure 25-7 in the textbook

Description:

_____

_____

_____

252

Chapter **25** **The Neonatal Brain**

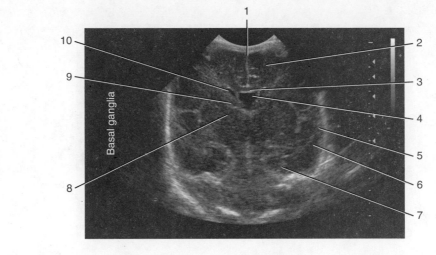

Figure 25-8 in the textbook

1	_____	6	_____
2	_____	7	_____
3	_____	8	_____
4	_____	9	_____
5	_____	10	_____

Description:

_____

_____

_____

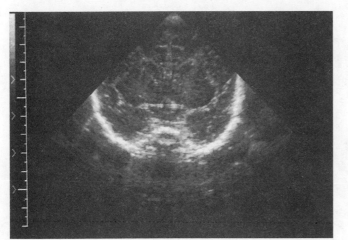 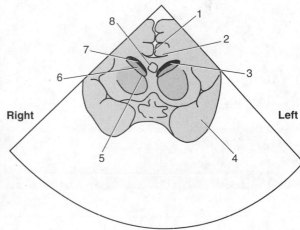

Figure 25-9 in the textbook

1	_____	5	_____
2	_____	6	_____
3	_____	7	_____
4	_____	8	_____

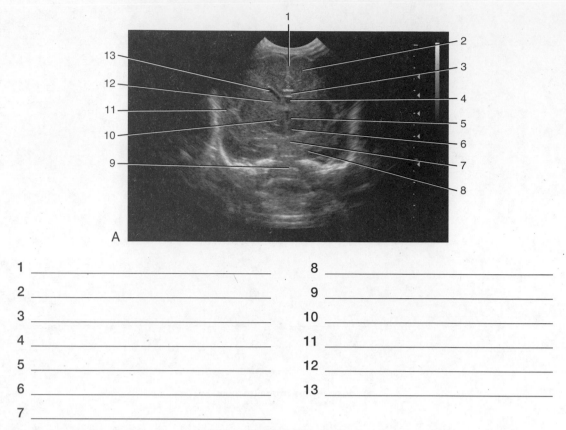

1	_____	8	_____
2	_____	9	_____
3	_____	10	_____
4	_____	11	_____
5	_____	12	_____
6	_____	13	_____
7	_____		

Figure 25-11A in the textbook

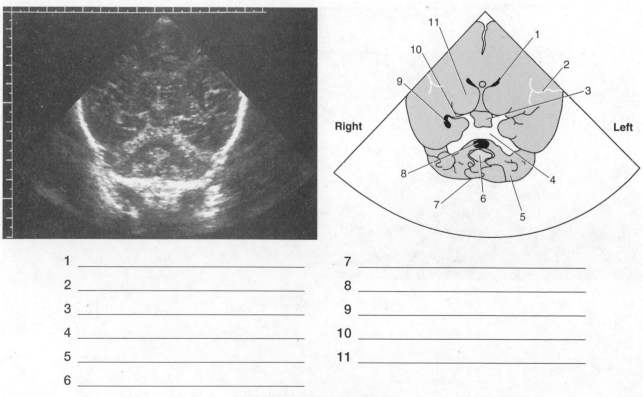

1	_____	7	_____
2	_____	8	_____
3	_____	9	_____
4	_____	10	_____
5	_____	11	_____
6	_____		

Figure 25-13 in the textbook

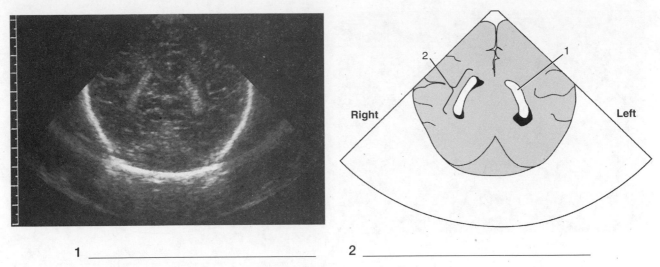

1 _____   2 _____

Figure 25-14 in the textbook

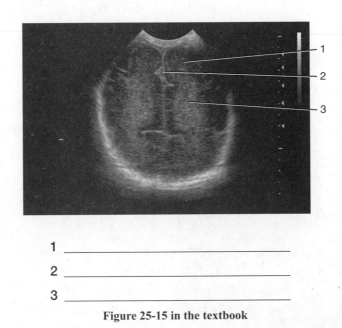

1 _____

2 _____

3 _____

Figure 25-15 in the textbook

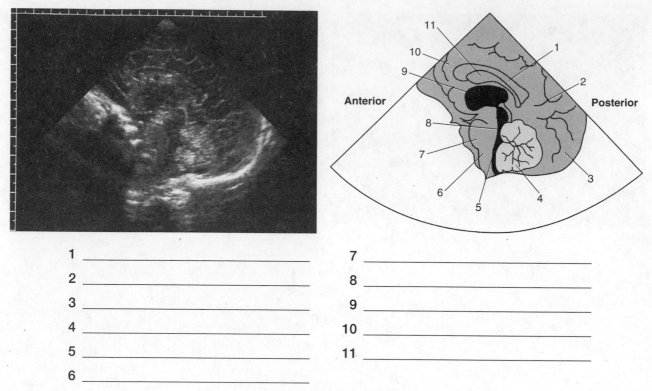

1	_____	7	_____
2	_____	8	_____
3	_____	9	_____
4	_____	10	_____
5	_____	11	_____
6	_____		

Figure 25-17 in the textbook

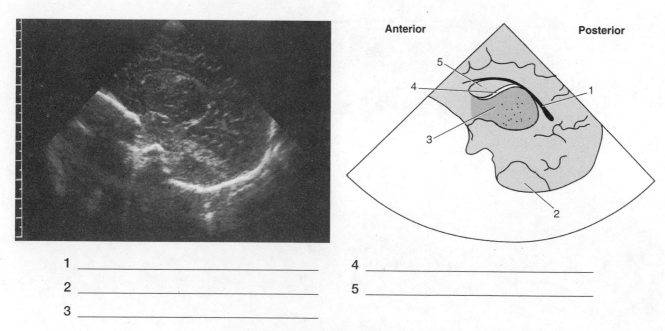

1	_____	4	_____
2	_____	5	_____
3	_____		

Figure 25-18 in the textbook

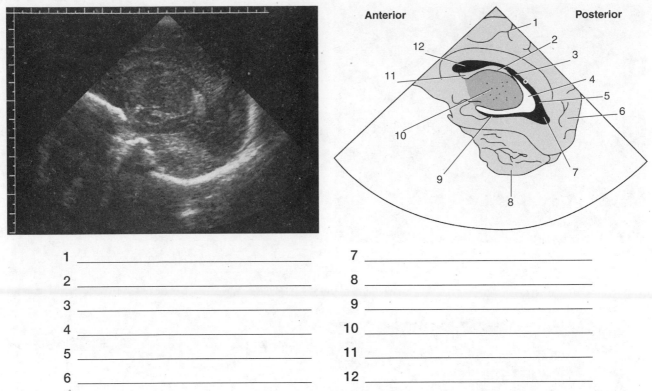

Anterior **Posterior**

1 _____   7 _____
2 _____   8 _____
3 _____   9 _____
4 _____   10 _____
5 _____   11 _____
6 _____   12 _____

Figure 25-19 in the textbook

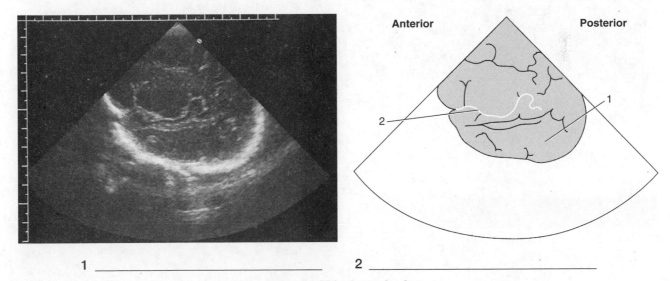

Anterior **Posterior**

1 _____   2 _____

Figure 25-20 in the textbook

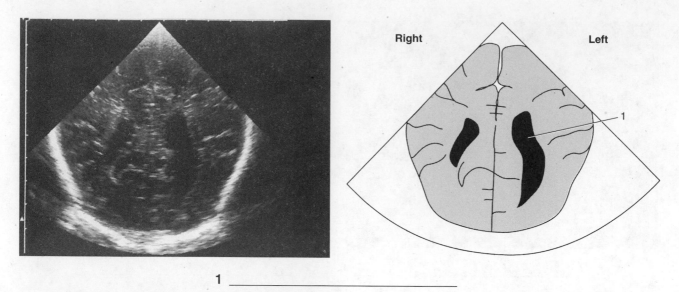

Right   Left

1 _____

Figure 25-21 in the textbook

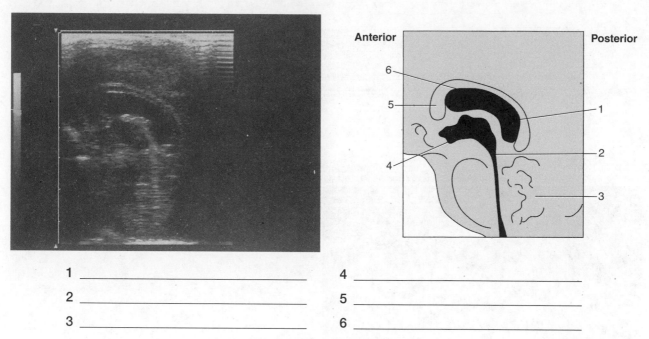

Anterior   Posterior

1 _____   4 _____

2 _____   5 _____

3 _____   6 _____

Figure 25-22 in the textbook

V. CHAPTER SUBHEADINGS EXERCISE

1. Convert each chapter subheading into a question; for example, change "Gross Anatomy" to "What is the gross anatomy of the neonatal brain?" Write the answer to each question in a short paragraph in your notebook. Exchange answers with your lab partner and check each other's work. Refer back to the textbook for further information and explanation.

2. What questions about the chapter do you still have? Write your questions in your notebook.

VI. CHAPTER EVALUATION EXERCISE

Use a fresh sheet of notebook paper. Based on your work with the chapter and its accompanying laboratory assignments, identify three concepts you believe are the most important. You may draw from any of the assignments you've already completed in the previous pages, including learning objectives, anatomy and physiology, images, or chapter subheadings. Include a detailed rationale in your answers.

Answer the questions below. Refer to page 372 for the answers.

Multiple Choice

1. The anterior fontanelle is commonly referred to as the
   a. hot spot.
   b. cold spot.
   c. soft spot.
   d. bony cover.

2. Over past decades, what has been the primary imaging method for evaluation of the neonatal brain?
   a. MRI
   b. CT
   c. Sonography
   d. Nuclear medicine

3. _____ are the cells that create brain activity.
   a. Protons
   b. Neurons
   c. Neutrons
   d. Gyri

4. The largest component of the central nervous system is the
   a. cerebrum.
   b. cerebellum.
   c. frontal lobe.
   d. basal ganglia.

5. The brain stem is also known as the
   a. pons.
   b. midbrain.
   c. hindbrain.
   d. thalami.

6. The function of the cerebellum is to
   a. make cerebrospinal fluid.
   b. provide balance and equilibrium to the body.
   c. provide functions such as speech and memory.
   d. store the brain's sensory receptors.

7. The _____ is responsible for speech, memory, voluntary movement, logical reasoning, and emotional response.
   a. cerebellum
   b. cerebrum
   c. brain stem
   d. choroid plexus

8. Which of the following is NOT a normal variant of the premature neonatal brain?
   a. Asymmetry of the lateral ventricles is a common variant.
   b. The lateral ventricles can measure any size and be normal.
   c. The left ventricle is generally larger than the right ventricle.
   d. Ventricular size can vary among infants.

9. This is an anechoic, fluid-filled space between the anterior horns of the lateral ventricles.
   a. Cavum septum vergae
   b. Cavum septum pellucidum
   c. Posterior ventricle
   d. Fourth ventricle

10. This area is highly susceptible to hemorrhage in the premature infant. It comprises a fine network of blood vessels and neural tissue.
    a. Germinal matrix
    b. Corpus callosum
    c. Cerebellum
    d. Periventricular white matter

The Thyroid and Parathyroid Glands **26**

I. MEMORIZATION EXERCISE

1. Write the key words in your notebook or on note cards. Write the words on one side of the notepaper and then write the definitions on the opposite side of the page or on the back of the paper. If using note cards, write the key word on the front and the definition on the back. *This step should be completed before the lab session begins.*

Memorize the key word definitions silently for 5 minutes, then work with a lab partner and identify the words you still need help with. List the words here. Add additional rows if needed.

II. COMPREHENSION EXERCISE

Work with a lab partner to complete this exercise. You will need to write in your notebook. First, change each objective into a question.

> *Example: "Describe the physiology of the thyroid and parathyroid glands" becomes "What is the physiology of the thyroid and parathyroid glands?"*

Next, write a short answer to the question just created.

> *Example: "The thyroid is essential to normal growth and development, and regulates basal metabolism, including blood calcium concentrations, through three hormones— triiodothyronine (T_3), thyroxine (T_4), and calcitonin. The parathyroids are four small glands embedded in the thyroid, two on each side, that also help maintain blood calcium concentrations."*

Highlight or circle any part of your answers about which you are unsure, and check the answers in your textbook. If you are still unsure of the answers, put a question mark next to the answer(s) for the review session of the lab.

III. APPLICATION OF ANATOMY AND PHYSIOLOGY EXERCISE

1. Label the diagram of the cross sectional thyroid gland and proximal structures as shown in the figure below. Colorize the structures. Refer to Figure 26-1 to check and correct your answers.

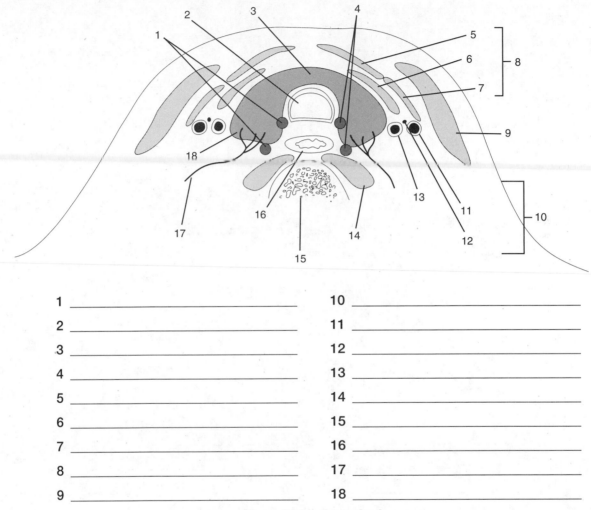

1	_____	10	_____
2	_____	11	_____
3	_____	12	_____
4	_____	13	_____
5	_____	14	_____
6	_____	15	_____
7	_____	16	_____
8	_____	17	_____
9	_____	18	_____

Figure 26-1 in the textbook

2. Label the diagram of the thyroid gland and proximal structures as shown in the figure below. Colorize the structures. Refer to Figure 26-2 to check and correct your answers.

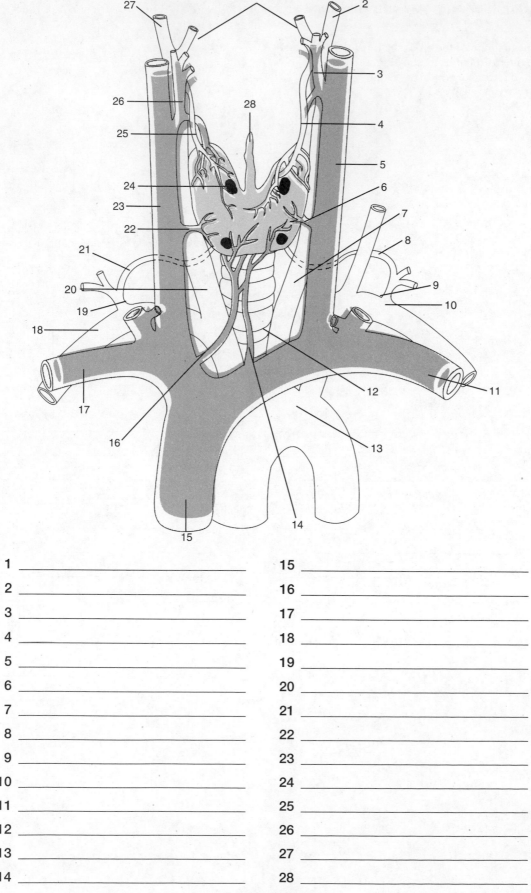

Figure 26-2 in the textbook

1	_____	15	_____
2	_____	16	_____
3	_____	17	_____
4	_____	18	_____
5	_____	19	_____
6	_____	20	_____
7	_____	21	_____
8	_____	22	_____
9	_____	23	_____
10	_____	24	_____
11	_____	25	_____
12	_____	26	_____
13	_____	27	_____
14	_____	28	_____

3. Write two or three summary sentences about the physiology of the thyroid and parathyroid. Ask your lab partner to check your work. Now check your work against the physiology section in the textbook. What else can you add to your description?

IV. IMAGE ANALYSIS EXERCISE

Work on the following figures with a lab partner, a group or independently. The goal is to label correctly all of the sketches and carefully compare the sketch with the sonographic image.

For each sonographic image, write a brief observation that could be "presented" to your instructor, a clinical sonographer, or a sonologist. Please review the section from Chapter 1 on How to Describe Ultrasound Findings. Remember that you want to:

- **recognize** normal echo patterns so you can identify abnormal presentations,
- **document** differences in echo pattern appearance, and
- **describe** differences in echo pattern appearance using sonographic terminology.

For each image, your assessment should include (1) the view of each major structure (axial or longitudinal; note: these are not the scanning planes) and (2) structures identified in the image with correct sonographic appearance description and measurements if shown.

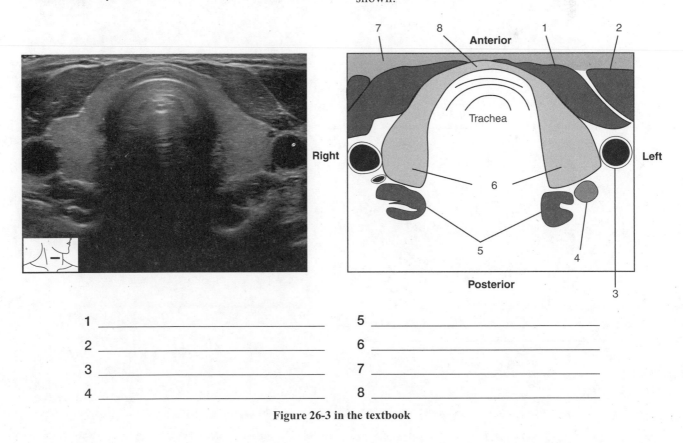

Figure 26-3 in the textbook

1 _____   5 _____

2 _____   6 _____

3 _____   7 _____

4 _____   8 _____

Description: _____

_____

_____

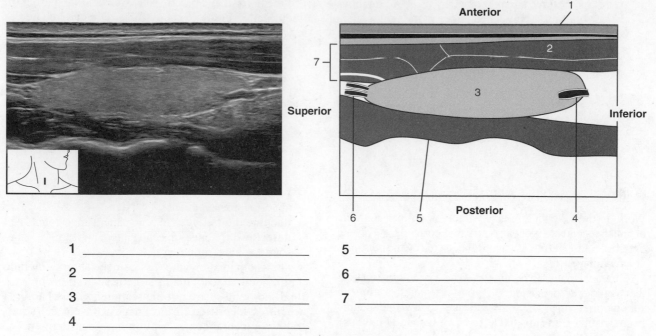

Figure 26-4 in the textbook

1 _____   5 _____

2 _____   6 _____

3 _____   7 _____

4 _____

Description: _____

_____

_____

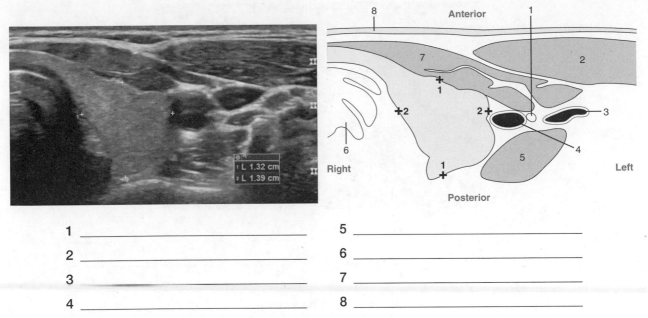

1	_____	5	_____
2	_____	6	_____
3	_____	7	_____
4	_____	8	_____

Figure 26-5 in the textbook

Description: _____

_____

_____

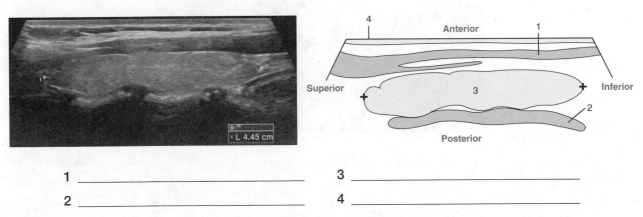

| 1 | _____ | 3 | _____ |
| 2 | _____ | 4 | _____ |

Figure 26-6 in the textbook

Description: _____

_____

_____

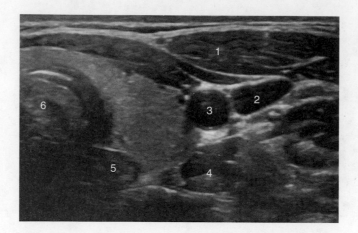

1 _____	4 _____
2 _____	5 _____
3 _____	6 _____

Figure 26-9 in the textbook

Description: _____

_____

_____

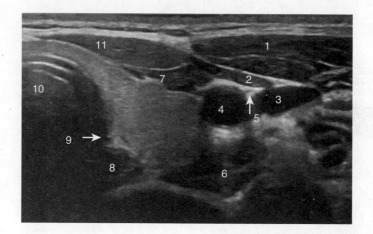

1 _____	7 _____
2 _____	8 _____
3 _____	9 _____
4 _____	10 _____
5 _____	11 _____
6 _____	

Figure 26-11 in the textbook

Description: _____

_____

_____

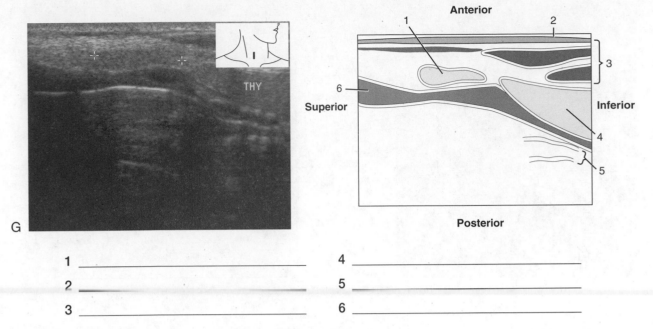

Figure 26-15 in the textbook

1 _____   4 _____

2 _____   5 _____

3 _____   6 _____

Description: _____

_____

_____

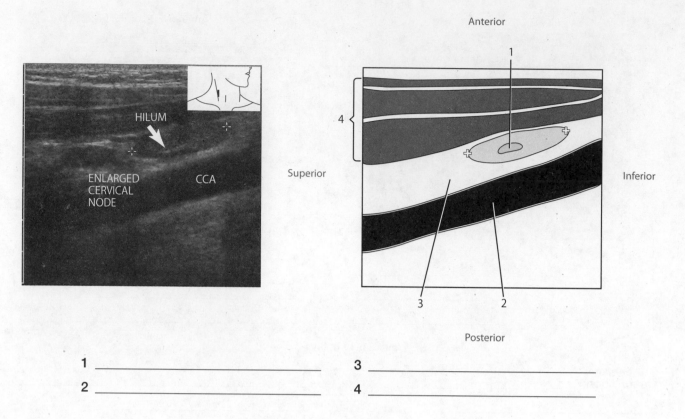

Figure 26-23 in the textbook

1 _____   3 _____
2 _____   4 _____

Description: _____
_____
_____

V. CHAPTER SUBHEADINGS EXERCISE

1. Convert each chapter subheading into a question; for example, change "Normal Variants" to "What is the normal sonographic appearance of the normal thyroid?" Write the answer to each question in a short paragraph in your notebook. Exchange answers with your lab partner and check each other's work. Refer back to the textbook for further information and explanation.

2. What questions do you still have about the chapter? Write your questions in your notebook.

VI. CHAPTER EVALUATION EXERCISE

Use a fresh sheet of notebook paper. Based on your work with the chapter and its accompanying laboratory assignments, identify three concepts you believe are the most important. You may draw from any of the assignments you've already completed in the previous pages, including learning objectives, anatomy and physiology, images, or chapter subheadings. Include a detailed rationale in your answers.

Answer the questions below. Refer to page 372 for the answers.

Multiple Choice

1. Which of the following muscles does not comprise the strap muscles?
   a. Infrahyoid
   b. Sternocleidomastoid
   c. Sternohyoid
   d. Omohyoid

2. Which statement is NOT true about the thyroid gland?
   a. It is located below the larynx.
   b. It is a gland with low vascularity.
   c. A pyramidal lobe is present in approximately 10% of the population.
   d. It has a saddlebag appearance in cross section.

3. Which of the following falls in the normal range for the thyroid gland in the average adult?
   a. 5 cm in length, 1.5 cm in AP diameter, 2 cm in width
   b. 4 cm in length, 3 cm in AP diameter, 2 cm in width
   c. 3 cm in length, 3 cm in AP diameter, 2 cm in width
   d. 6 cm in length, 2 cm in AP diameter, 3 cm in width

4. How many lobes make up the thyroid gland?
   a. Two
   b. Four
   c. Six
   d. Eight

5. The lobes of the thyroid gland are connected by the
   a. pyramidal lobe.
   b. trachea.
   c. isthmus.
   d. parathyroid.

6. The longus colli neck muscle(s) are located
   a. anterior in the neck, superficial to the larynx, trachea, and thyroid.
   b. anterolateral to the thyroid.
   c. laterally in the neck, deep to the sternocleidomastoid.
   d. posterior to the thyroid.

7. All of the following increase the thyroid volume EXCEPT:
   a. Increased body weight
   b. Increased amounts of iodine intake
   c. Acute hepatitis
   d. Increased age

8. The size and shape of thyroids vary; which measurement is used to determine if the thyroid is enlarged?
   a. Length
   b. Anteroposterior diameter
   c. Width
   d. Volume

9. Which of the following hormones controls the amount of thyroid secretion?
   a. TSH
   b. T3
   c. T4
   d. Calcitonin

10. Which of the following hormones prevents hypercalcemia?
    a. Thyroxine
    b. Triiodothyronine
    c. Calcitonin
    d. Thyrotropin

I. MEMORIZATION EXERCISE

1. Write the key words in your notebook or on note cards. Write the words on one side of the notepaper and then write the definitions on the opposite side of the page or on the back of the paper. If using note cards, write the key word on the front and the definition on the back. *This step should be completed before the lab session begins.*

   Memorize the key word definitions silently for 5 minutes, then work with a lab partner and identify the words you still need help with. List the words here. Add additional rows if needed.

II. COMPREHENSION EXERCISE

1. Work with a lab partner to complete this exercise. You will need to write in your notebook. First, change each objective into a question.

   Example: "Describe the location of anatomy related to the breast" becomes "Where is anatomy of the breast located?"

Next, write a short answer to the question just created.

   Example: "The breast is anterior to the pectoralis major, serratus, and external oblique muscles. Each breast is lateral to the sternum and medial to the axilla. The layers of the breast, moving from anterior to posterior, are skin, subcutaneous fat, glandular tissue, subcutaneous fat, and posterior muscle."

Highlight or circle any part of your answers about which you are unsure, and check the answers in your textbook. If you are still unsure of the answers, put a question mark next to the answer(s) for the review session of the lab.

III. APPLICATION OF ANATOMY AND PHYSIOLOGY EXERCISE

1. Label the breast; include each structure's orientation in the body (either vertical, horizontal, vertical oblique, or horizontal oblique). Ask your lab partner to critique your work.

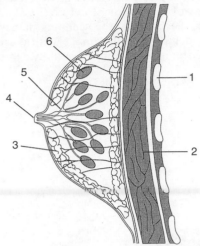

Figure 27-1 in the textbook

1	_____
2	_____
3	_____
4	_____
5	_____
6	_____

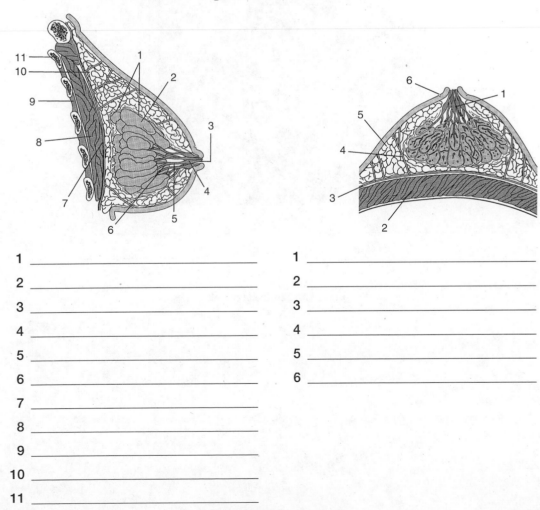

1	_____
2	_____
3	_____
4	_____
5	_____
6	_____
7	_____
8	_____
9	_____
10	_____
11	_____

1	_____
2	_____
3	_____
4	_____
5	_____
6	_____

Figure 27-3 in the textbook

IV. IMAGE ANALYSIS EXERCISE

Work on the following figures with your lab partner. It's your choice! You can label all the sketches at once, then go back and label each image with your lab partner, or label an image and its accompanying sketch at the same time. Either way, the goal is to label correctly all of the sketches and carefully compare the sketch with the sonographic image.

For each sonographic image, write a brief observation that could be "presented" to your instructor, a clinical sonographer, or a sonologist. Please review the section from Chapter 1 on How to Describe Ultrasound Findings. Remember that you want to:

- **differentiate** abnormal echo patterns from normal echo patterns,
- **document** any differences in echo pattern appearance, and
- **describe** any difference in echo pattern appearance using sonographic terminology.

For each image, your assessment should include (1) the view of each major structure (axial or longitudinal; note: these are not the scanning planes) and (2) structures identified in the image with correct sonographic appearance description and measurements if shown.

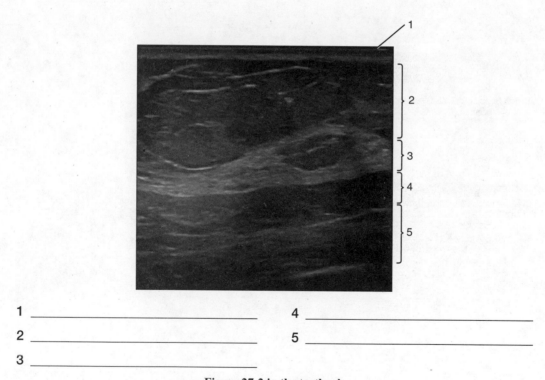

1 _____   4 _____

2 _____   5 _____

3 _____

Figure 27-2 in the textbook

Chapter **27 Breast Sonography**

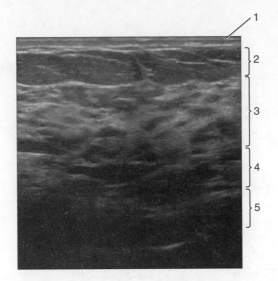

1 _____	4 _____
2 _____	5 _____
3 _____	

Figure 27-4 in the textbook

Description: _____

_____

_____

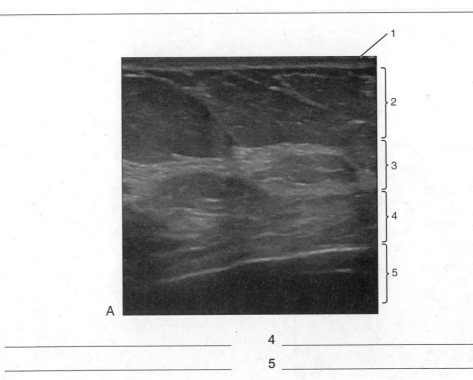

A

1 _____	4 _____
2 _____	5 _____
3 _____	

Figure 27-5A in the textbook

Description: _____

_____

_____

Chapter **27** **Breast Sonography**

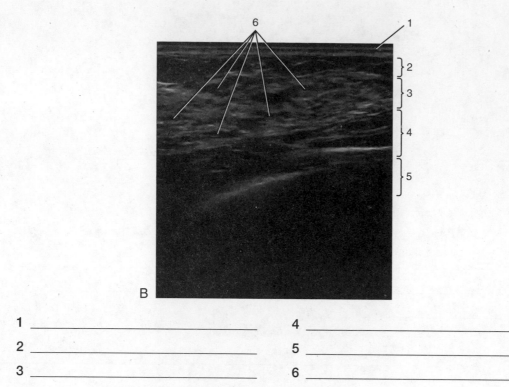

Figure 27-5B in the textbook

1 _____	4 _____
2 _____	5 _____
3 _____	6 _____

Description: _____

_____

_____

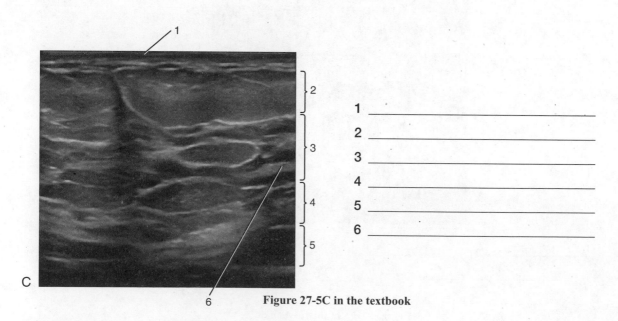

Figure 27-5C in the textbook

1 _____
2 _____
3 _____
4 _____
5 _____
6 _____

Description: _____

_____

_____

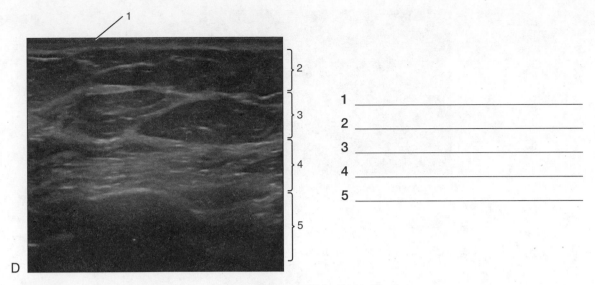

Figure 27-5D in the textbook

1 _____

2 _____

3 _____

4 _____

5 _____

Description: _____
_____
_____

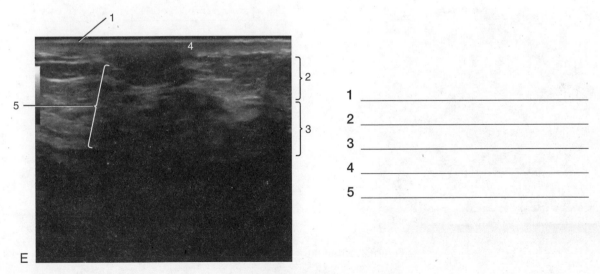

Figure 27-5E in the textbook

1 _____

2 _____

3 _____

4 _____

5 _____

Description: _____
_____
_____

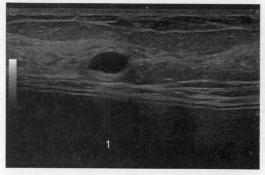

1 _____

Figure 27-6A in the textbook

Description: _____
_____
_____

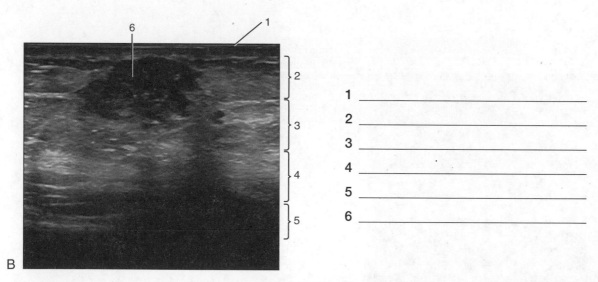

1 _____
2 _____
3 _____
4 _____
5 _____
6 _____

Figure 27-6B in the textbook

Description: _____
_____
_____

Chapter **27** **Breast Sonography**

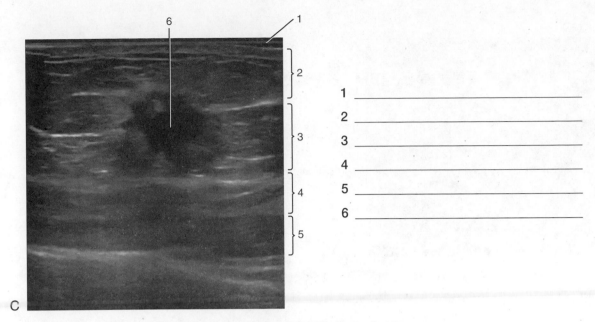

C

Figure 27-6C in the textbook

1 _____

2 _____

3 _____

4 _____

5 _____

6 _____

Description: _____

_____

_____

D

(Courtesy GE Imaging, Waukesha, Wisconsin.)

1 _____   4 _____

2 _____   5 _____

3 _____   6 _____

Figure 27-6D in the textbook

Description: _____

_____

_____

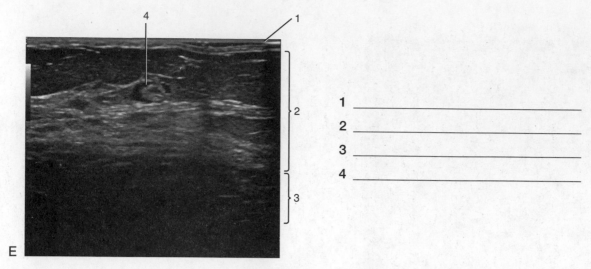

E

Figure 27-6E in the textbook

1 _____

2 _____

3 _____

4 _____

Description: _____

_____

_____

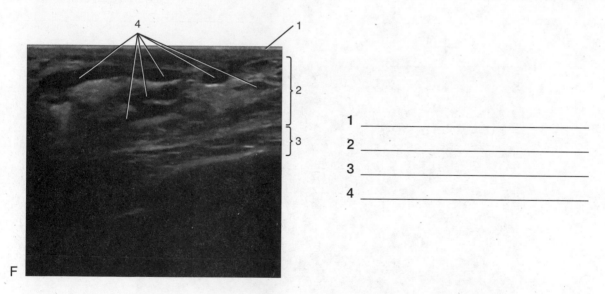

F

Figure 27-6F in the textbook

1 _____

2 _____

3 _____

4 _____

Description: _____

_____

_____

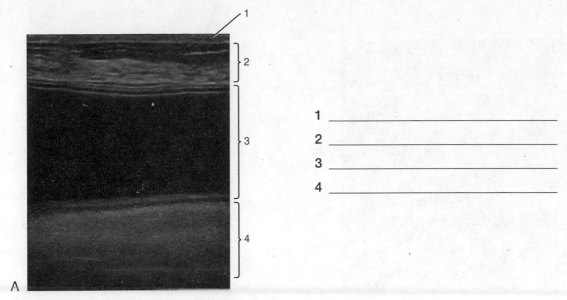

Figure 27-7A in the textbook

Description: _____

_____

_____

1 _____
2 _____
3 _____
4 _____

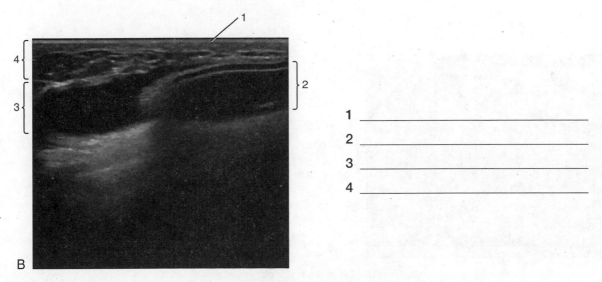

Figure 27-7B in the textbook

Description: _____

_____

_____

1 _____
2 _____
3 _____
4 _____

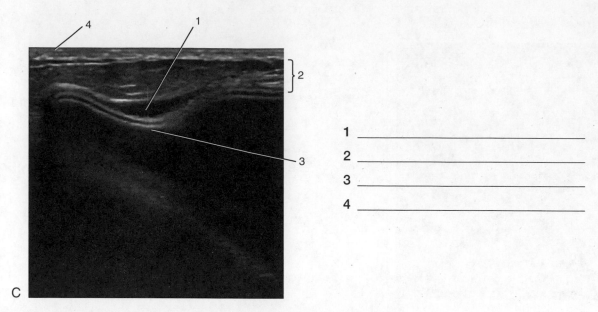

Figure 27-7C in the textbook

1	_____
2	_____
3	_____
4	_____

Description: _____

_____

_____

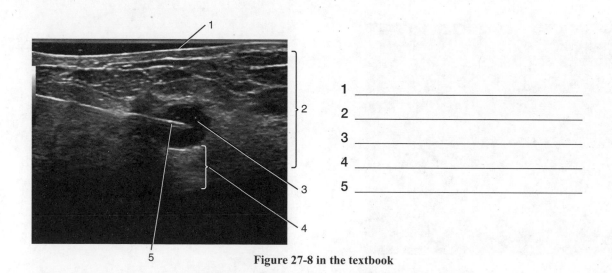

Figure 27-8 in the textbook

1	_____
2	_____
3	_____
4	_____
5	_____

Description: _____

_____

_____

V. CHAPTER SUBHEADINGS EXERCISE

1. Convert each chapter subheading into a question; for example, change "Gross Anatomy" to "What is the gross anatomy of the breast?" Write the answer to each question in a short paragraph in your notebook. Exchange answers with your lab partner and check each other's work. Refer back to the textbook for further information and explanation.

2. What questions do you still have about the chapter? Write your questions in your notebook.

VI. CHAPTER EVALUATION EXERCISE

Use a fresh sheet of notebook paper. Based on your work with the chapter and its accompanying laboratory assignments, identify three concepts you believe are the most important. You may draw from any of the assignments you've already completed in the previous pages, including learning objectives, anatomy and physiology, images, or chapter subheadings. Include a detailed rationale in your answers.

Answer the questions below. Refer to page 372 for the answers.

Matching

_____ 1. Contains glandular tissues, ducts, and connective tissues

_____ 2. Hormone that stimulates contraction of the lactiferous ducts for milk secretion

_____ 3. Hormone that stimulates the development of breast lobules and alveoli for lactation

_____ 4. Ampulla for each lactiferous duct near the nipple where milk can be stored

_____ 5. Grape-shaped secretory portions of a gland

_____ 6. Contains skin and subcutaneous fat

_____ 7. Hormone that stimulates breast tissue development

_____ 8. Ducts in the parenchyma of the breast that secrete milk after pregnancy

_____ 9. Glandular tissue elements within mammary lobules

_____ 10. Contains retromammary fat, muscle, and deep connective tissues

a. Acini
b. Alveoli
c. Estrogen
d. Lactiferous ducts
e. Mammary layer
f. Montgomery's glands
g. Oxytocin
h. Progesterone
i. Retromammary layer
j. Subcutaneous layer

Scrotal and Penile Sonography 28

I. MEMORIZATION EXERCISE

1. Write the key words in your notebook or on note cards. Write the words on one side of the notepaper and then write the definitions on the opposite side of the page or on the back of the paper. If using note cards, write the key word on the front and the definition on the back. *This step should be completed before the lab session begins.*

    Memorize the key word definitions silently for 5 minutes, then work with a lab partner and identify the words you still need help with. List the words here. Add additional rows if needed.

II. COMPREHENSION EXERCISE

Work with a lab partner to complete this exercise. You will need to write in your notebook. First, change each objective into a question.

> *Example: "Describe the normal size of the testicles" becomes "What is the normal size of the testicles?"*

Next, write a short answer to the question just created.

> *Example: "The normal adult testicle measures approximately 3 to 5 cm (1.5 to 2 inches) in length, 2 to 3 cm (1 inch) in anterior-to-posterior dimension, and 2 to 3 cm (1 inch) in width. The adult testicular volume is approximately 25 mL and weighs 10 to 15 g. It is only one-fifth of that volume before puberty and decreases in size with advancing age."*

Highlight or circle any part of your answers about which you are unsure, and check the answers in your textbook. If you are still unsure of the answers, put a question mark next to the answer(s) for the review session of the lab.

1. Label the structures of the male pelvis. Below the diagram, write a few sentences about the physiology of the structures shown. Check your work against the physiology section of the textbook. What did you miss?

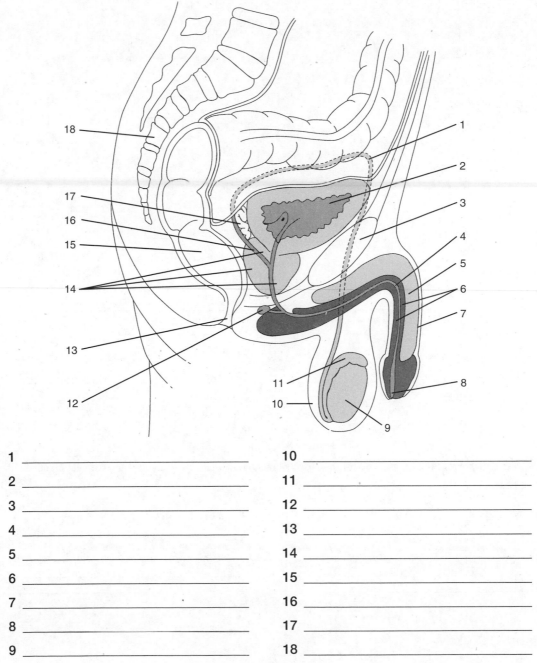

1 _____	10 _____
2 _____	11 _____
3 _____	12 _____
4 _____	13 _____
5 _____	14 _____
6 _____	15 _____
7 _____	16 _____
8 _____	17 _____
9 _____	18 _____

Figure 28-1 in the textbook

Description:

_____

_____

_____

2. Label cross-section of the scrotum. Below the diagram, write a few sentences about the physiology of the structures shown. Check your work against the physiology section of the textbook. What did you miss?

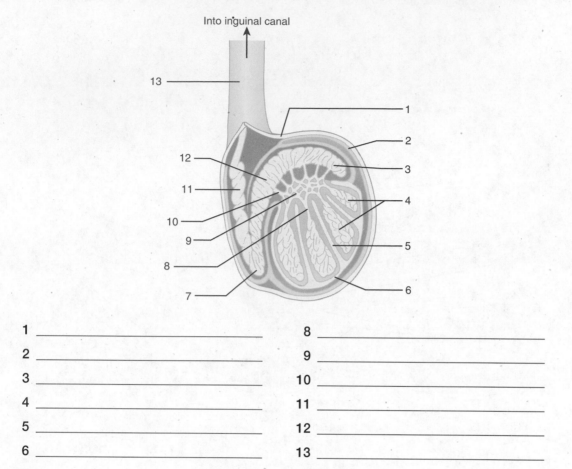

Figure 28-3 in the textbook

(From Walls R.M., Hockberger R.S., Gasuche-Hill M. Rosen's Emergency Medicine: Concepts and Clinical Practice, 9th ed, St. Louis, 2018, Elsevier.)

1	_____	8	_____
2	_____	9	_____
3	_____	10	_____
4	_____	11	_____
5	_____	12	_____
6	_____	13	_____
7	_____		

Description:

_____
_____
_____

3. Label the penile anatomy. Below the diagram, write a few sentences about the physiology of the structures shown. Check your work against the physiology section of the textbook. What did you miss?

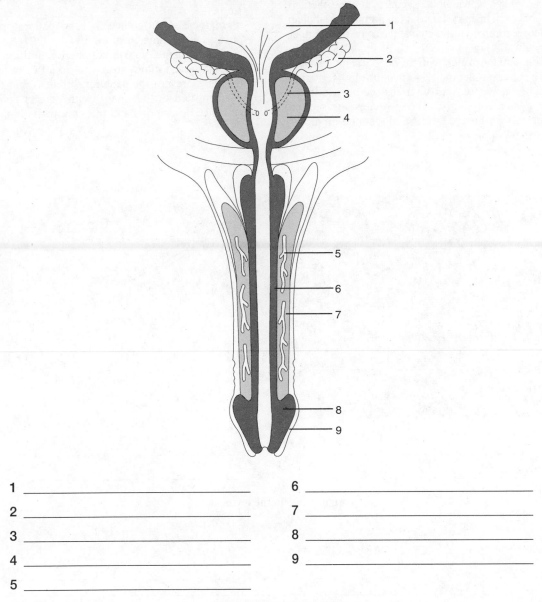

1 _____   6 _____

2 _____   7 _____

3 _____   8 _____

4 _____   9 _____

5 _____

Figure 28-6 in the textbook

Description:

_____

_____

_____

IV. IMAGE ANALYSIS EXERCISE

Work on the following figures with your lab partner. It's your choice! You can label all the sketches at once, then go back and label each image with your lab partner, or label an image and its accompanying sketch at the same time. Either way, the goal is to label correctly all of the sketches and carefully compare the sketch with the sonographic image.

For each sonographic image, write a brief observation that could be "presented" to your instructor, a clinical sonographer, or a sonologist. Please review the section from Chapter 1 on How to Describe Ultrasound Findings. Remember that you want to:

- **differentiate** abnormal echo patterns from normal echo patterns,
- **document** any differences in echo pattern appearance, and
- **describe** any difference in echo pattern appearance using sonographic terminology.

For each image, your assessment should include (1) the view of each major structure (axial or longitudinal; note: these are not the scanning planes) and (2) structures identified in the image with correct sonographic appearance description and measurements if shown.

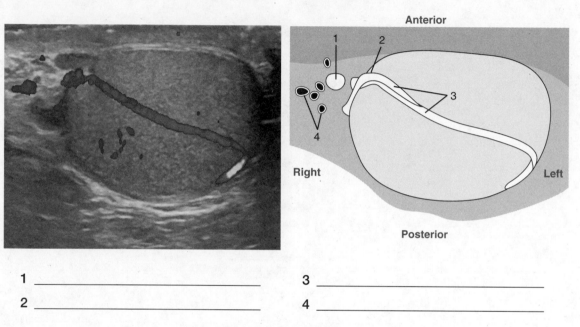

1 _____   3 _____

2 _____   4 _____

Figure 28-5 in the textbook

Description:

_____

_____

_____

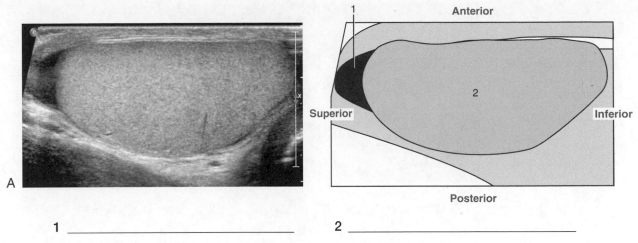

1 _____   2 _____

Figure 28-7A in the textbook

Description:

_____
_____
_____

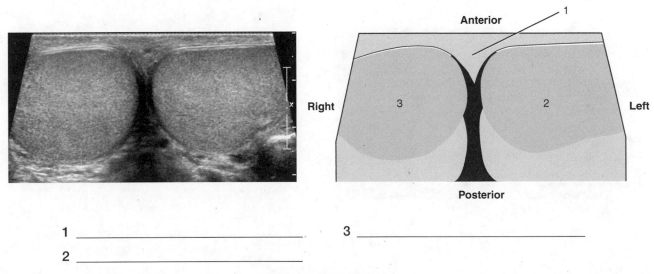

1 _____   3 _____

2 _____

Figure 28-8 in the textbook

Description:

_____
_____
_____

287

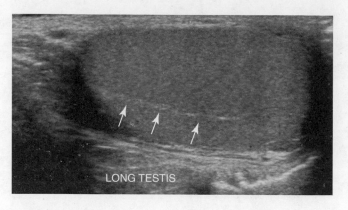

Arrows: _____

Figure 28-11 in the textbook

Description:

_____

_____

_____

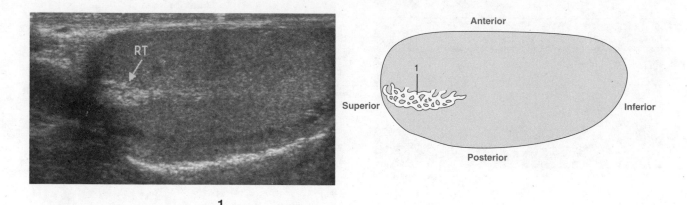

1 _____

Figure 28-13 in the textbook

Description:

_____

_____

_____

Chapter **28** **Scrotal and Penile Sonography**

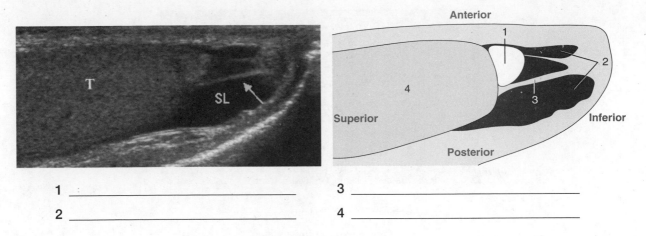

1 _____	3 _____
2 _____	4 _____

Figure 28-14 in the textbook

Description:

_____

_____

_____

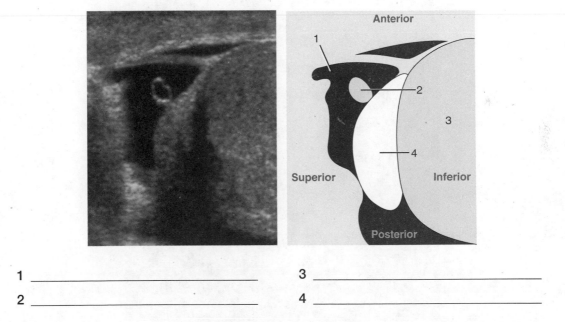

1 _____	3 _____
2 _____	4 _____

Figure 28-16 in the textbook

Description:

_____

_____

_____

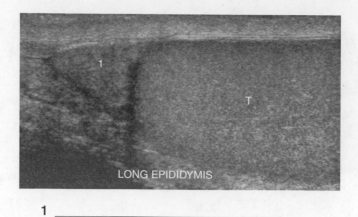

LONG EPIDIDYMIS

1 _____

Figure 28-17 in the textbook

Description:

_____

_____

_____

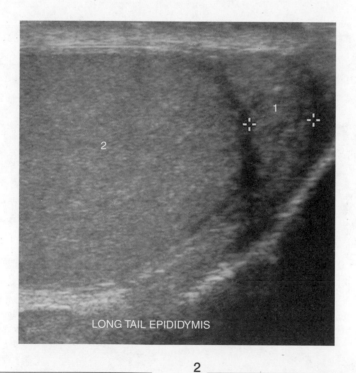

LONG TAIL EPIDIDYMIS

1 _____   2 _____

Figure 28-19 in the textbook

Description:

_____

_____

_____

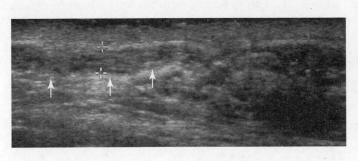
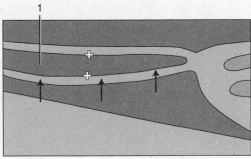

1 _____

Figure 28-21 in the textbook

Description:

_____

_____

_____

V. CHAPTER SUBHEADINGS EXERCISE

1. Convert each chapter subheading into a question; for example, change "Gross Anatomy" to "What is the gross anatomy of the penis and scrotum?" Write the answer to each question in a short paragraph in your notebook. Exchange answers with your lab partner and check each other's work. Refer back to the textbook for further information and explanation.
2. What questions do you still have about the chapter? Write your questions in your notebook.

VI. CHAPTER EVALUATION EXERCISE

Use a fresh sheet of notebook paper. Based on your work with the chapter and its accompanying laboratory assignments, identify three concepts you believe are the most important. You may draw from any of the assignments you've already completed in the previous pages, including learning objectives, anatomy and physiology, images, or chapter subheadings. Include a detailed rationale in your answers.

Answer the questions below. Refer to page 372 for the answers.

Multiple Choice

1. The remnant of what structure is known as the scrotal ligament?
   a. Tunica dartos
   b. Paradidymis
   c. Gubernaculum
   d. Buck's fascia

2. The scrotum is divided into two compartments: externally by _____ and internally by _____.
   a. Buck's fascia; tunica vaginalis
   b. Median raphe; tunica albuginea
   c. Darto's fascia, infundibuliform fascia
   d. Median raphe; tunica dartos

3. The cremaster muscle surrounds each testicle and performs what important function?
   a. Contractions control blood flow into erectile tissues.
   b. Contractions regulate internal temperature of testicles.
   c. Contractions help to control ejaculation.
   d. Contractions help testicles drop from inguinal canal into scrotum.

4. This dense, white fibrous tissue covers the testis and forms the mediastinum testis and interlobar septa:
   a. Tunica vaginalis
   b. Tunica albuginea
   c. Tunica vasculosa
   d. Tunica adventitia

5. The septa of the mediastinum radiate into the testicle and separate into how many lobules?
   a. 10–30
   b. 50–100
   c. 200–300
   d. 400–600

6. The epididymis is composed mostly of this single convoluted tube:
   a. Ductus epididymis
   b. Ductus deferens
   c. Ductus aberrans
   d. Seminiferous tubule

7. This structure is divided into globus major, corpus and globus minor:
   a. vas deferens
   b. scrotum
   c. Giraldes organ
   d. epididymis

8. The corpora cavernosa and corpus spongiosum are three cylindrical masses of tissue of what structure?
   a. Testis
   b. Epididymis
   c. Penis
   d. Pampiniform plexus

9. Sonographically, normal testicular parenchyma is homogeneous and similar in appearance to
   a. epididymis.
   b. pancreas.
   c. kidney.
   d. thyroid.

10. This is a network of fibrous connective tissue continuous with the tunica albuginea that invaginates the posterior aspect of the testis and encloses the rete testis:
    a. Pampiniform plexus
    b. Mediastinum testis
    c. Recurrent rami
    d. Tunica vaginalis

29 Pediatric Echocardiography

I. MEMORIZATION EXERCISE

1. Write the key words in your notebook or on note cards. Write the words on one side of the notepaper and then write the definitions on the opposite side of the page or on the back of the paper. If using note cards, write the key word on the front and the definition on the back. *This step should be completed before the lab session begins.*

   Memorize the key word definitions silently for 5 minutes, then work with a lab partner and identify the words you still need help with. List the words here. Add additional rows if needed.

II. COMPREHENSION EXERCISE

Work with a lab partner to complete this exercise. You will need to write in your notebook. First, change each objective into a question.

> *Example: "Name the chambers, great veins, and great arteries of the heart" becomes "What are the chambers, great veins, and great arteries of the heart?"*

Next, write a short answer to the question just created.

> *Example: "There are four chambers in the heart. The right atrium and right ventricle are connected by the tricuspid valve, which transports blood to the lungs, via a great artery—the pulmonary artery. The great veins that empty blood into the right atrium are the superior and inferior vena cavae. The left atrium and left ventricle are the remaining two chambers; they bring oxygenated blood from the lungs and ultimately to the rest of the body via the second great artery, the aorta. Oxygenated blood is returned to the left atrium via four pulmonary veins."*

Highlight or circle any part of your answers about which you are unsure, and check the answers in your textbook. If you are still unsure of the answers, put a question mark next to the answer(s) for the review session of the lab.

1. Label the transducer positions.

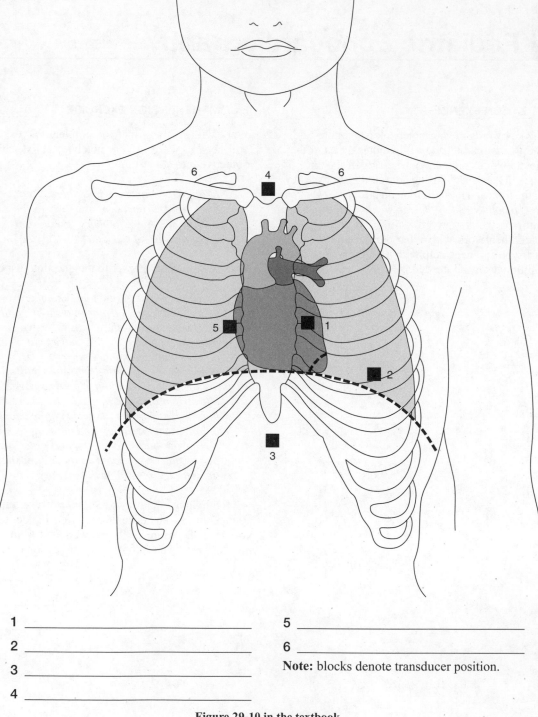

1 _____   5 _____

2 _____   6 _____

3 _____   **Note:** blocks denote transducer position.

4 _____

Figure 29-10 in the textbook

2. Label the neonatal heart.

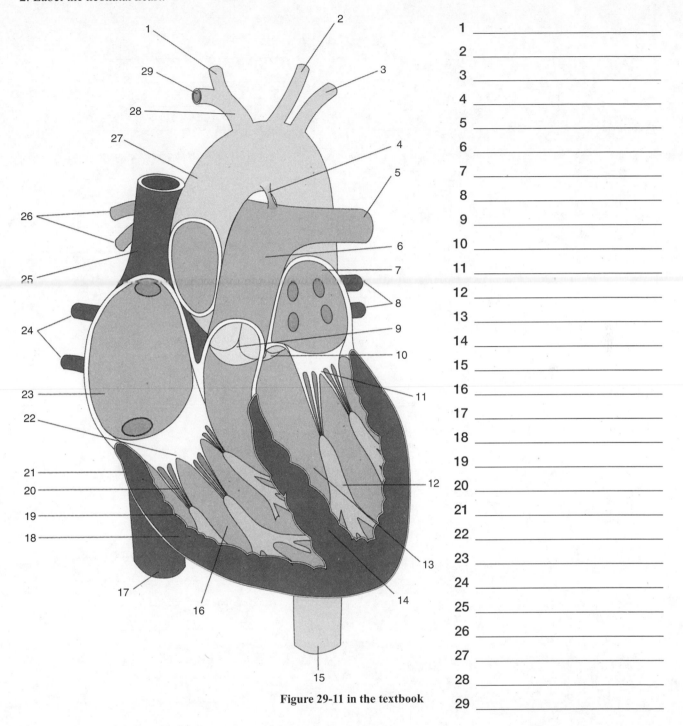

Figure 29-11 in the textbook

1 _____
2 _____
3 _____
4 _____
5 _____
6 _____
7 _____
8 _____
9 _____
10 _____
11 _____
12 _____
13 _____
14 _____
15 _____
16 _____
17 _____
18 _____
19 _____
20 _____
21 _____
22 _____
23 _____
24 _____
25 _____
26 _____
27 _____
28 _____
29 _____

3. Label the coronary arteries in the anterior view.

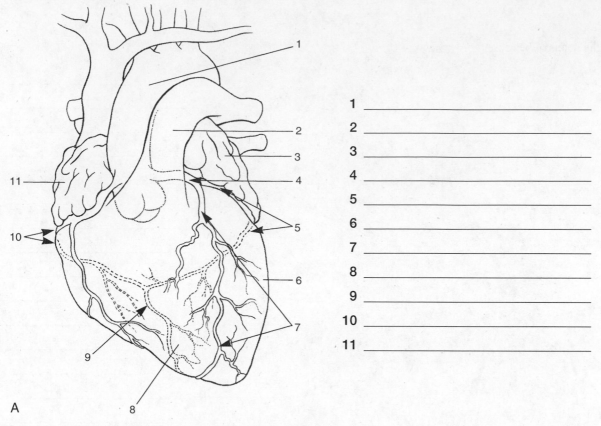

A

Coronary arteries and their positions on the heart, anterior view.

Figure 29-13A in the textbook

1 _____
2 _____
3 _____
4 _____
5 _____
6 _____
7 _____
8 _____
9 _____
10 _____
11 _____

4. Label the coronary arteries in the posterior view.

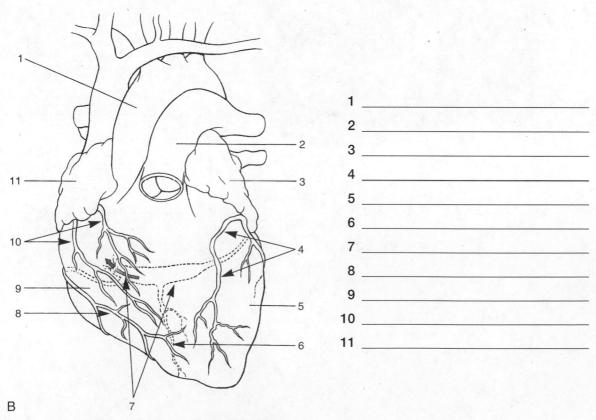

B

Cardiac veins and their positions on the heart, anterior view.

Figure 29-13B in the textbook

1 _____
2 _____
3 _____
4 _____
5 _____
6 _____
7 _____
8 _____
9 _____
10 _____
11 _____

5. Label the parts of the conduction system.

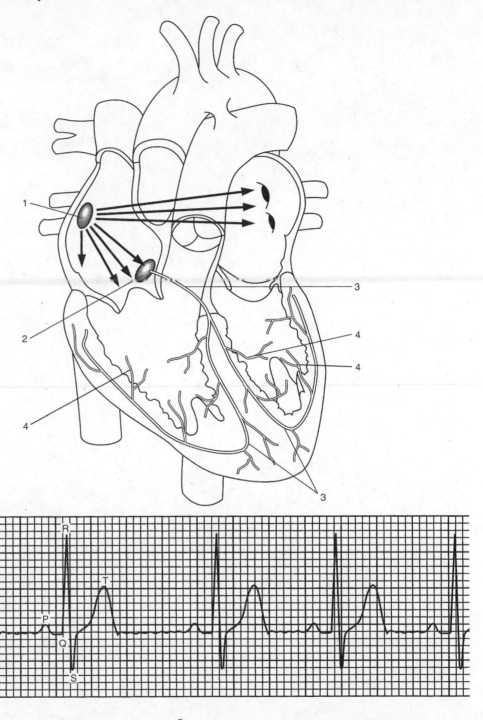

Figure 29-14 in the textbook

1 _____   3 _____

2 _____   4 _____

Description: _____

_____

_____

6. Label the heart anatomy visualized in each plane.

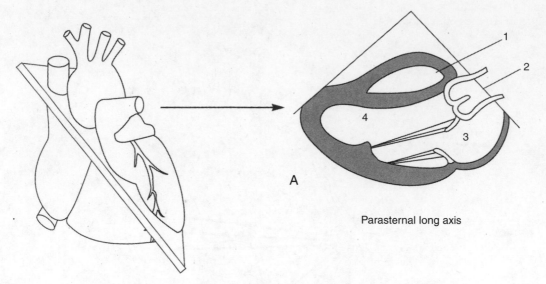

A

Parasternal long axis

Figure 29-15A in the textbook

Parasternal short axis

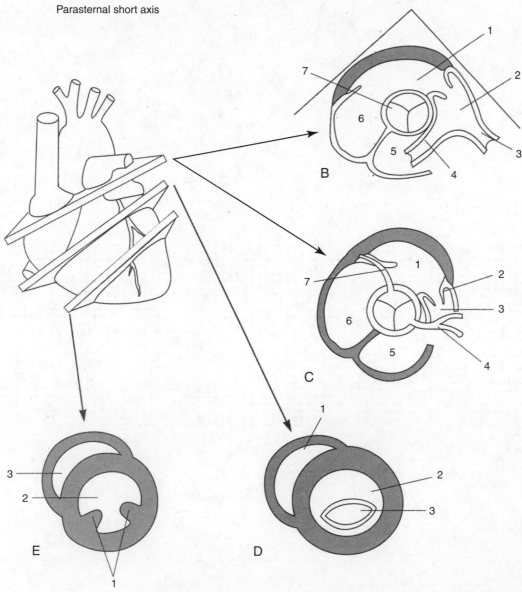

B

C

E

D

Figure 29-15B to E in the textbook

A

1 _____

2 _____

3 _____

4 _____

B

1 _____

2 _____

3 _____

4 _____

5 _____

6 _____

7 _____

C

1 _____

2 _____

3 _____

4 _____

5 _____

6 _____

7 _____

D

1 _____

2 _____

3 _____

E

1 _____

2 _____

3 _____

Figure 29-15A to E in the textbook

Description: _____

_____

_____

IV. IMAGE ANALYSIS EXERCISE

Work on the following figures with your lab partner. It's your choice! You can label all the sketches at once, then go back and label each image with your lab partner, or label an image and its accompanying sketch at the same time. Either way, the goal is to label correctly all of the sketches and carefully compare the sketch with the sonographic image.

For each sonographic image, write a brief observation that could be "presented" to your instructor, a clinical sonographer, or a sonologist. Please review the section from Chapter 1 on How to Describe Ultrasound Findings. Remember that you want to:

- **differentiate** abnormal echo patterns from normal echo patterns,
- **document** any differences in echo pattern appearance, and
- **describe** any difference in echo pattern appearance using sonographic terminology.

For each image, your assessment should include (1) the view of each major structure (axial or longitudinal; note: these are not the scanning planes) and (2) structures identified in the image with correct sonographic appearance description and measurements if shown.

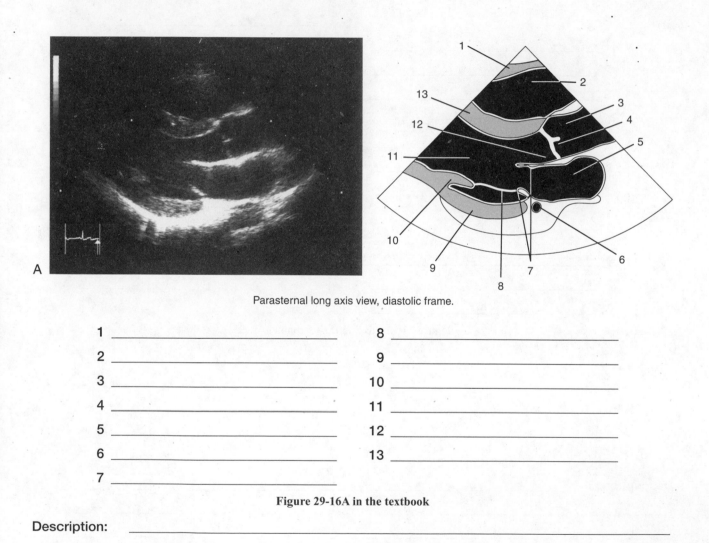

Parasternal long axis view, diastolic frame.

1 _____	8 _____
2 _____	9 _____
3 _____	10 _____
4 _____	11 _____
5 _____	12 _____
6 _____	13 _____
7 _____	

Figure 29-16A in the textbook

Description: _____

_____

_____

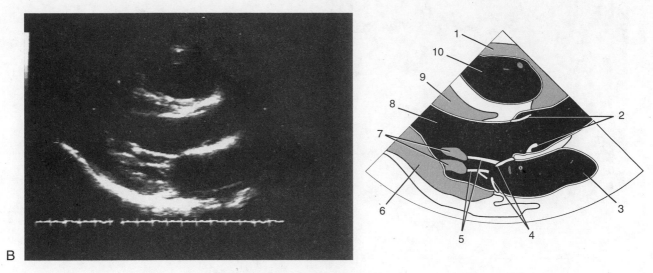

Parasternal long axis view, systolic frame.

1 _____	6 _____
2 _____	7 _____
3 _____	8 _____
4 _____	9 _____
5 _____	10 _____

Figure 29-16B in the textbook

Description: _____

_____

_____

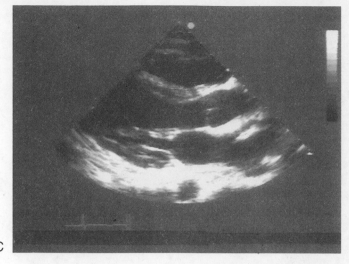

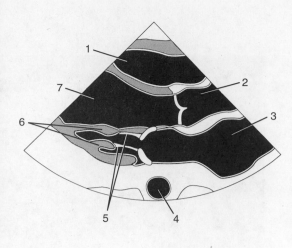

C

Parasternal long axis view, late diastolic frame.

1 _____   5 _____

2 _____   6 _____

3 _____   7 _____

4 _____

Figure 29-16C in the textbook

Description: _____

_____

_____

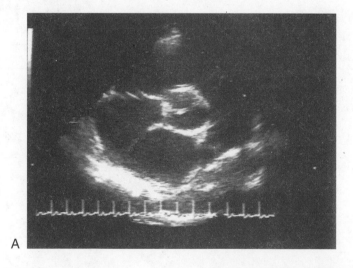

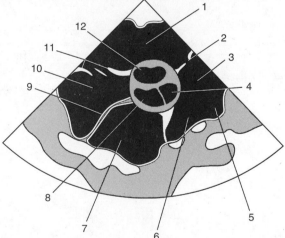

A

Closed aortic valve, parasternal short axis section.

1 _____   7 _____

2 _____   8 _____

3 _____   9 _____

4 _____   10 _____

5 _____   11 _____

6 _____   12 _____

Figure 29-21A in the textbook

Chapter **29** **Pediatric Echocardiography**

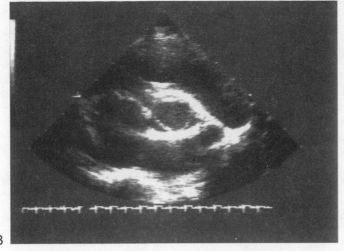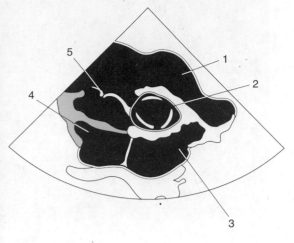

B

Open aortic valve, parasternal short axis section.

1 _____   4 _____

2 _____   5 _____

3 _____

Figure 29-21B in the textbook

Description: _____
_____
_____

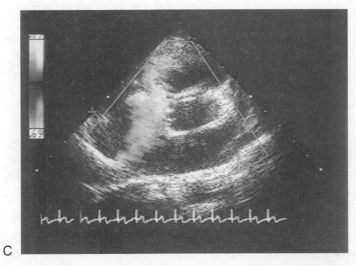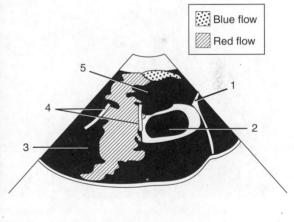

C

Flow through the tricuspid valve.

1 _____   4 _____

2 _____   5 _____

3 _____

Figure 29-21C in the textbook

Description: _____
_____
_____

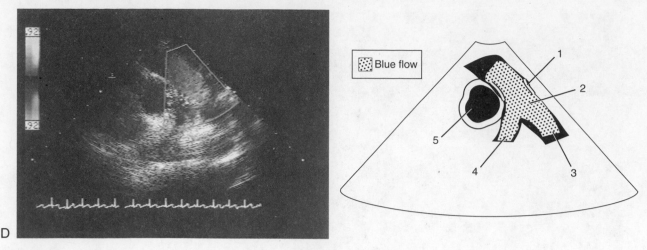

Flow through the pulmonary valve.

1 _____   4 _____

2 _____   5 _____

3 _____

Figure 29-21D in the textbook

Description: _____
_____
_____

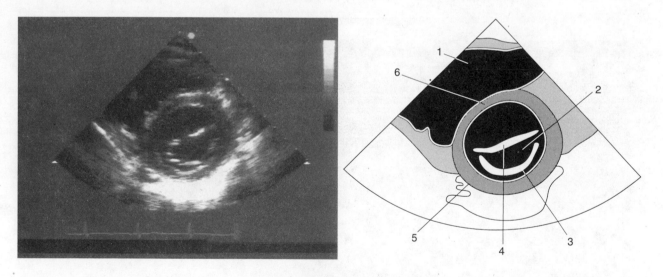

Mitral valve, short axis plane.

1 _____   4 _____

2 _____   5 _____

3 _____   6 _____

Figure 29-22, top, in the textbook

Description: _____
_____
_____

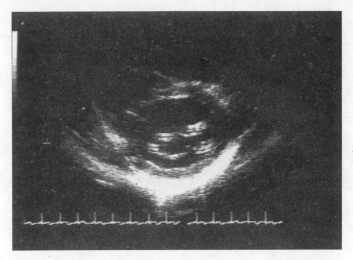
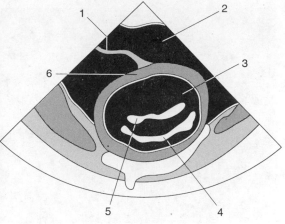

Mitral valve, short axis plane.

1 _____   4 _____
2 _____   5 _____
3 _____   6 _____

Figure 29-22, bottom, in the textbook

Description: _____

_____

_____

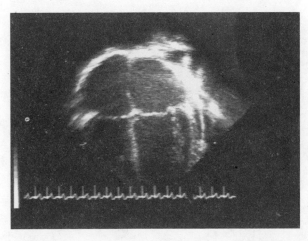
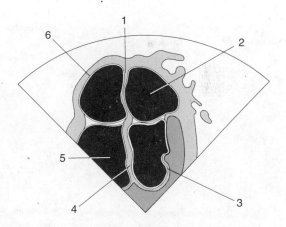

Apical four-chamber sections.

1 _____   4 _____
2 _____   5 _____
3 _____   6 _____

Figure 29-25A, top, in the textbook

Description: _____

_____

_____

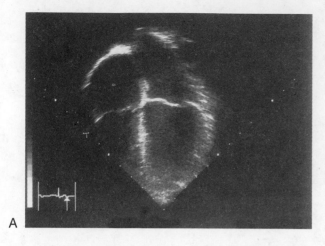

A

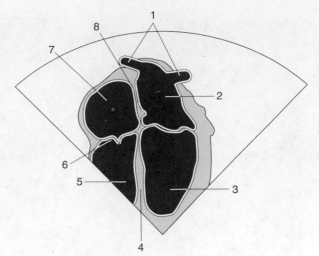

Color flow Doppler of the mitral valve.

1 _____   5 _____
2 _____   6 _____
3 _____   7 _____
4 _____   8 _____

Figure 29-25A, bottom, in the textbook

Description: _____

_____

_____

B

[] Red flow

1 _____   4 _____
2 _____   5 _____
3 _____

Figure 29-25B in the textbook

Description: _____

_____

_____

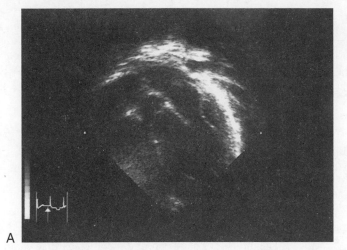
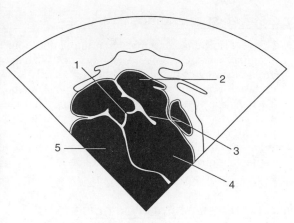

Apical long axis sections.

1 _____ 4 _____

2 _____ 5 _____

3 _____

Figure 29-26A, top, in the textbook

Description: _____

_____

_____

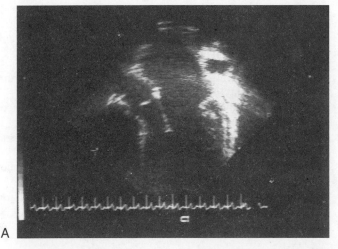
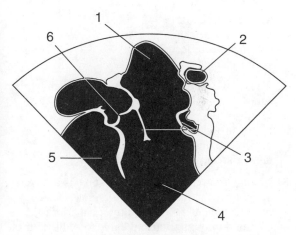

Apical long axis view with color flow.

1 _____ 4 _____

2 _____ 5 _____

3 _____ 6 _____

Figure 29-26A, bottom, in the textbook

Description: _____

_____

_____

V. CHAPTER SUBHEADINGS EXERCISE

1. Convert each chapter subheading into a question; for example, change "Gross Anatomy" to "What is the gross anatomy of the pediatric heart?" Briefly answer each question in a short paragraph in your notebook. Exchange answers with your lab partner and check each other's work. Refer back to the textbook for further information and explanation.
2. What questions do you still have about the chapter? Write your questions in your notebook.

VI. CHAPTER EVALUATION EXERCISE

Use a fresh sheet of notebook paper. Based on your work with the chapter and its accompanying laboratory assignments, identify three concepts you believe are the most important. You may draw from any of the assignments you've already completed in the previous pages, including learning objectives, anatomy and physiology, images, or chapter subheadings. Include a detailed rationale in your answers.

Answer the questions below. Refer to page 372 for the answers.

Multiple Choice

1. Which fetal shunt connects the umbilical vein to the IVC?
   a. Foramen ovale
   b. Ductus venosus
   c. Ductus arteriosus
   d. Eustachian valve

2. The truncus arteriosus divides into which two structures?
   a. Aorta and pulmonary artery
   b. Aorta and SVC
   c. Tricuspid and mitral valve
   d. Mitral and aortic valve

3. The function of the eustachian valve is to divert
   a. oxygenated blood across foramen ovale.
   b. deoxygenated blood to umbilical arteries
   c. blood through tricuspid valve to right ventricle.
   d. blood directly to ductus arteriosus.

4. Normal orientation of the abdominal organs and position of the heart is termed
   a. situs inversus.
   b. situs ambiguus.
   c. situs totalis.
   d. situs solitus.

5. The heart apex pointed to the patient's left chest is termed
   a. dextroposition.
   b. levoposition.
   c. levocardia.
   d. dextrocardia.

6. The most anterior chamber of the heart is the
   a. right atrium.
   b. right ventricle.
   c. left atrium.
   d. left ventricle.

7. The moderator band is found in which cardiac chamber?
   a. Right atrium
   b. Right ventricle
   c. Left atrium
   d. Left ventricle

8. Which structure is considered the pacemaker of the heart?
   a. Atrioventricular (AV) node
   b. Bundle of His
   c. Right and left bundle branches
   d. Sinoatrial (SA) node

9. Which transducer would provide superior detail of the premature infant heart?
   a. 12–8 MHz phased or vector array
   b. 6–3 MHz curved linear array
   c. 5–2 MHz phased or vector array
   d. 12–9 MHz sequential linear array

10. Which of the following is considered normal cardiac anatomy?
    a. Atrioventricular and ventriculoarterial discordance
    b. Atrioventricular discordance and ventriculoarterial concordance
    c. Atrioventricular and ventriculoarterial concordance
    d. Atrioventricular concordance and ventriculoarterial discordance

30 Adult Echocardiography

I. MEMORIZATION EXERCISE

1. Write the key words in your notebook or on note cards. Write the words on one side of the notepaper and then write the definitions on the opposite side of the page or on the back of the paper. If using note cards, write the key word on the front and the definition on the back. *This step should be completed before the lab session begins.*

   Memorize the key word definitions silently for 5 minutes, then work with a lab partner and identify the words you still need help with. List the words here. Add additional rows if needed.

Next, write a short answer to the question just created.

> *Example: "The heart sits within the thoracic cavity, posterior to the sternum and adjacent to the right and left lungs in the mediastinum. The heart sits within a sac called the pericardium. The heart sits at a slight angle, with its lower tip, or apex, pointed to the left of midline. The apex is more inferior and anterior than the base of the heart, where the pulmonary artery and aorta are located."*

Highlight or circle any part of your answers about which you are unsure, and check the answers in your textbook. If you are still unsure of the answers, put a question mark next to the answer(s) for the review session of the lab.

II. COMPREHENSION EXERCISE

1. Work with a lab partner to complete this exercise. You will need to write in your notebook. First, change each objective into a question.

   > *Example: "Describe the location of the heart in the chest" becomes "Where is the heart located in the chest?"*

1. Label the external structures and location of the heart in the thoracic cavity as shown in the figure below. Color the structures. Below your drawing, write two or three summary sentences on the physiology of the heart. Compare your summary with the physiology section of the textbook..

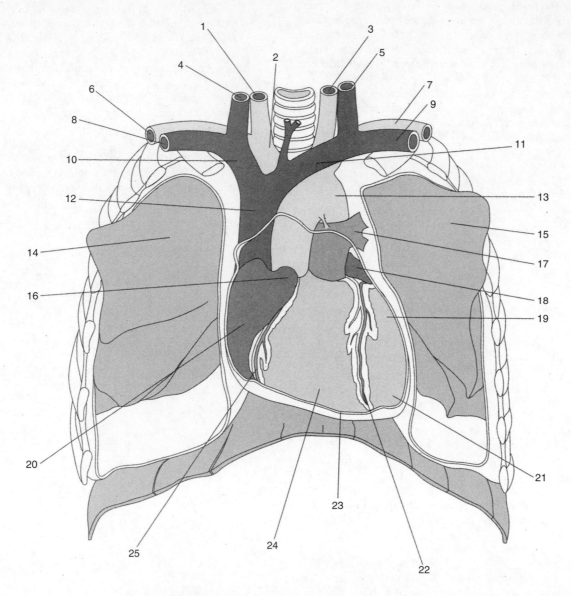

Figure 30-1 in the textbook Answer blanks are on following page.

1 _____   14 _____

2 _____   15 _____

3 _____   16 _____

4 _____   17 _____

5 _____   18 _____

6 _____   19 _____

7 _____   20 _____

8 _____   21 _____

9 _____   22 _____

10 _____   23 _____

11 _____   24 _____

12 _____   25 _____

13 _____

Figure 30-1 in the textbook

Physiology

_____

_____

_____

_____

_____

_____

_____

_____

2. Label the internal structures of the heart and its chambers and vessels. Color the structures.

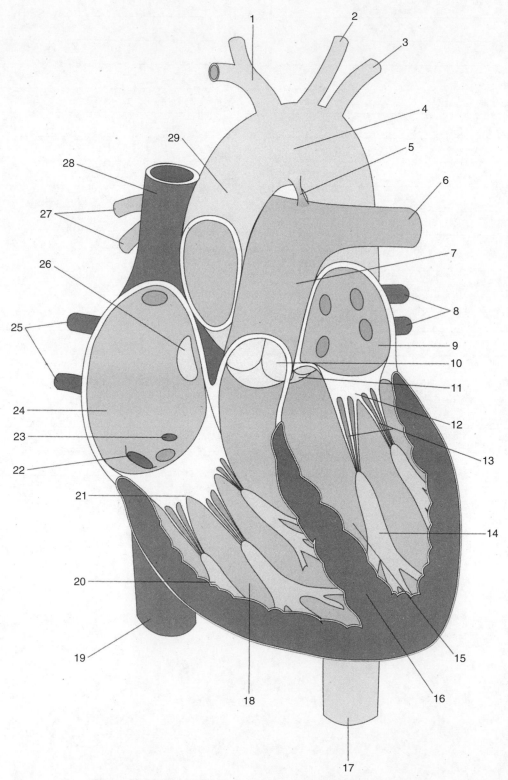

Figure 30-2 in the textbook Answer blanks are on following page.

1	_____	16	_____
2	_____	17	_____
3	_____	18	_____
4	_____	19	_____
5	_____	20	_____
6	_____	21	_____
7	_____	22	_____
8	_____	23	_____
9	_____	24	_____
10	_____	25	_____
11	_____	26	_____
12	_____	27	_____
13	_____	28	_____
14	_____	29	_____
15	_____		

Figure 30-2 in the textbook

3. Label the structures of the normal ECG showing the QRS complex.

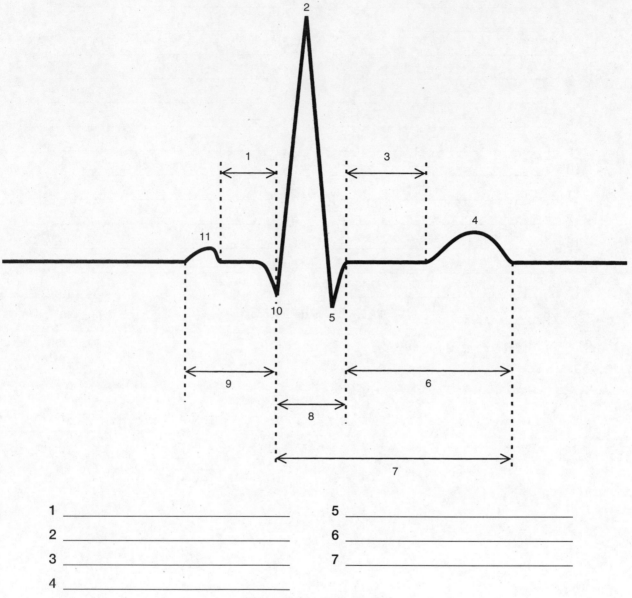

1 _____   5 _____

2 _____   6 _____

3 _____   7 _____

4 _____

Figure 30-7 in the textbook

IV. IMAGE ANALYSIS EXERCISE

Work on the following figures with a lab partner, a group or independently. The goal is to label correctly all of the sketches and carefully compare the sketch with the sonographic image.

For each sonographic image, write a brief observation that could be "presented" to your instructor, a clinical sonographer, or a sonologist. Please review the section from Chapter 1 on How to Describe Ultrasound Findings. Remember that you want to:

- **Recognize** normal echo patterns, so you can identify abnormal presentations
- **Document** differences in echo pattern appearance, and
- **Describe** differences in echo pattern appearance using sonographic terminology

For each image, your assessment should include (1) the view of each major structure (axial or longitudinal) and (2) structures identified in the image with correct sonographic appearance description and measurements if shown.

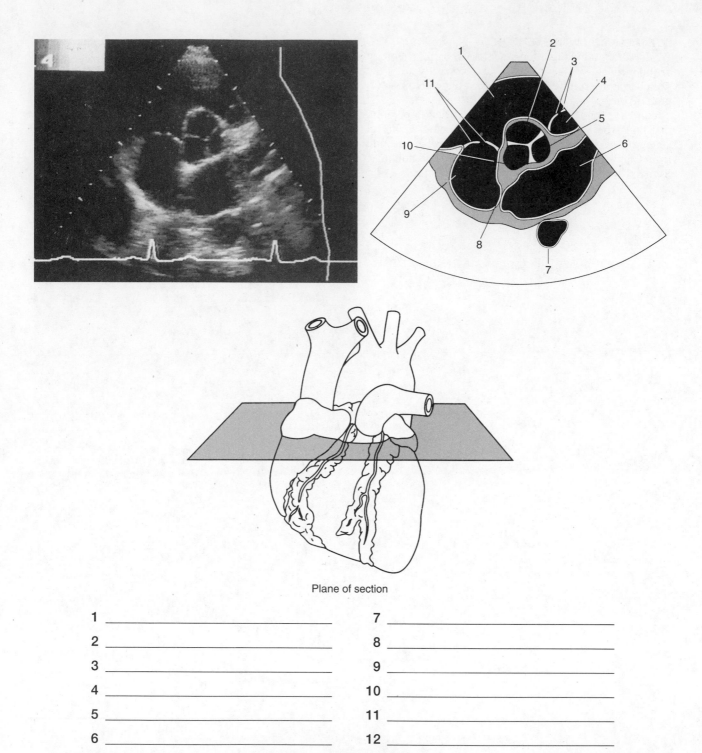

Plane of section

1	_____	7	_____
2	_____	8	_____
3	_____	9	_____
4	_____	10	_____
5	_____	11	_____
6	_____	12	_____

Figure 30-8 in the textbook

Description:

_____

_____

_____

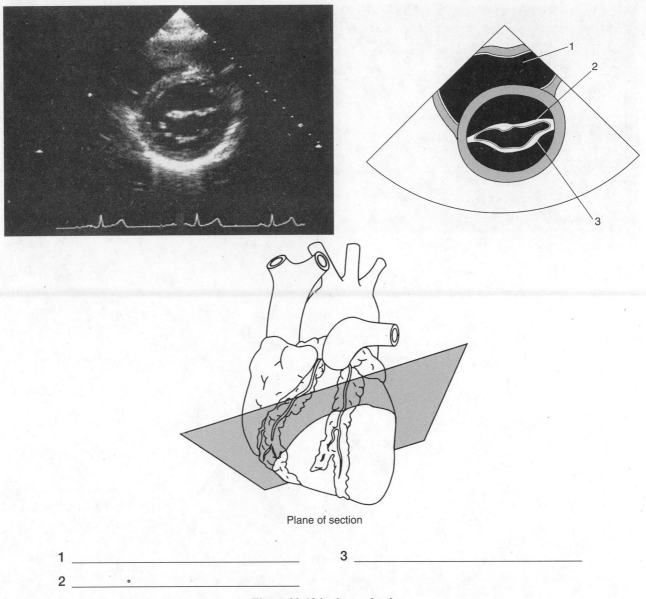

Plane of section

1 _____   3 _____

2 _____

Figure 30-12 in the textbook

Description:

_____

_____

_____

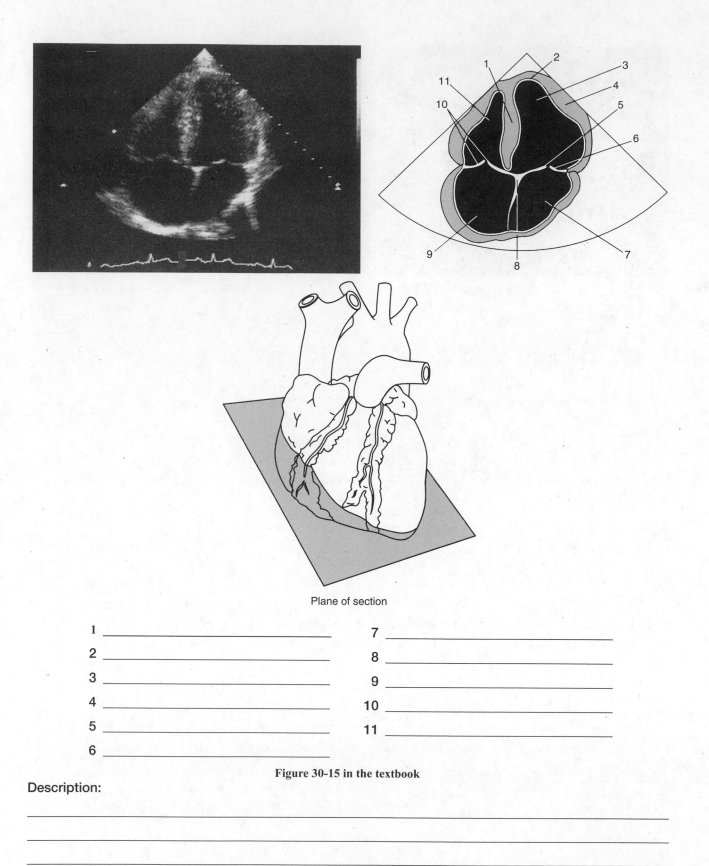

Plane of section

1 _____   7 _____

2 _____   8 _____

3 _____   9 _____

4 _____   10 _____

5 _____   11 _____

6 _____

Figure 30-15 in the textbook

Description:

_____

_____

_____

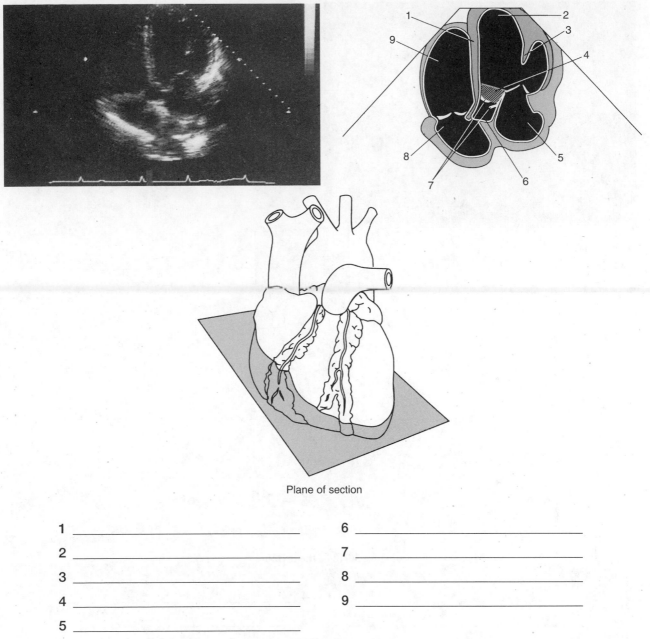

Plane of section

1 _____	6 _____
2 _____	7 _____
3 _____	8 _____
4 _____	9 _____
5 _____	

Figure 30-17 in the textbook

Description:

_____

_____

_____

Chapter **30** **Adult Echocardiography**

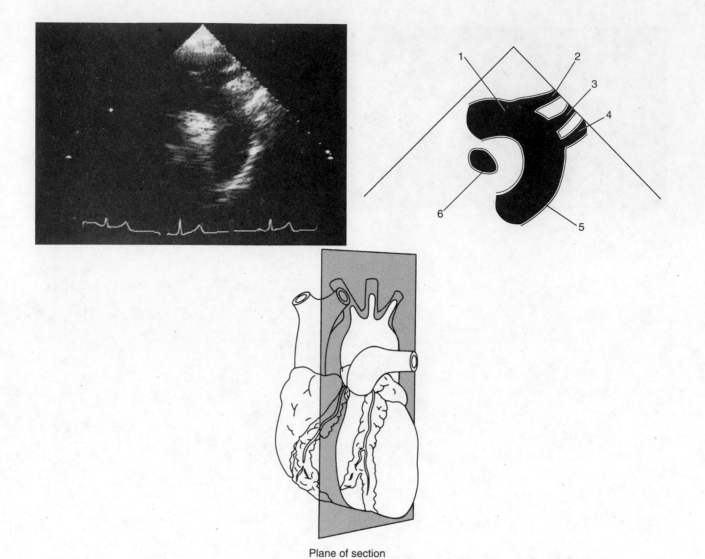

Plane of section

Figure 30-18 in the textbook

1 _____   4 _____

2 _____   5 _____

3 _____   6 _____

Description:

_____

_____

_____

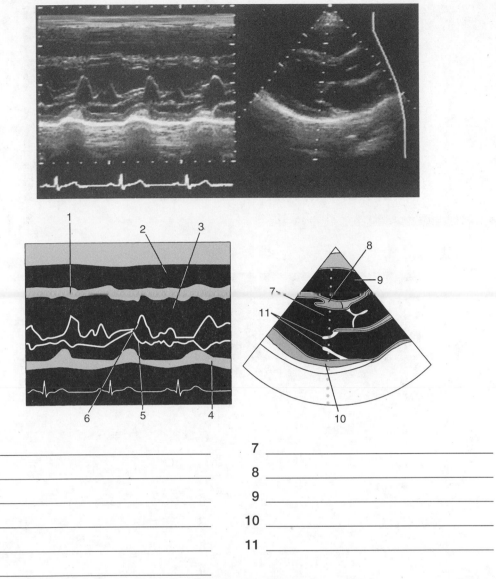

1	_____	7	_____
2	_____	8	_____
3	_____	9	_____
4	_____	10	_____
5	_____	11	_____
6	_____		

Figure 30-21 in the textbook

Description:

_____

_____

_____

_____

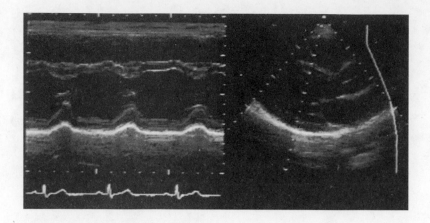

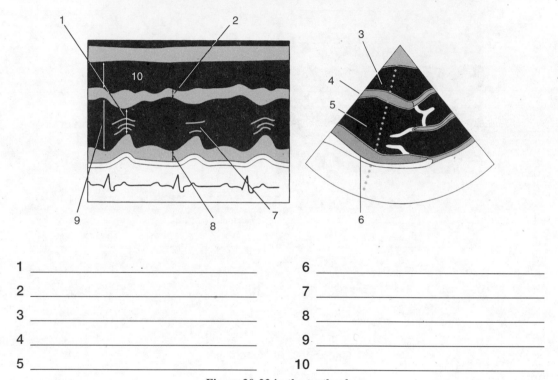

1	_____	6	_____
2	_____	7	_____
3	_____	8	_____
4	_____	9	_____
5	_____	10	_____

Figure 30-23 in the textbook

Description:

_____

_____

_____

V. CHAPTER SUBHEADINGS EXERCISE

1. Convert each chapter subheading into a question; for example, change "Gross Anatomy" to "What is the gross anatomy of the adult heart?" Briefly answer each question in a short paragraph in your notebook. Exchange answers with your lab partner and check each other's work. Refer back to the textbook for further information and explanation.
2. What questions do you still have about the chapter? Write your questions in your notebook.

VI. CHAPTER EVALUATION EXERCISE

Use a fresh sheet of notebook paper. Based on your work with the chapter and its accompanying laboratory assignments, identify three concepts you believe are the most important. You may draw from any of the assignments you've already completed in the previous pages, including learning objectives, anatomy and physiology, images, or chapter subheadings. Include a detailed rationale in your answers.

Answer the questions below. Refer to page 372 for the answers.

Multiple Choice

1. Which major vessel do the two major coronary arteries arise from?
   a. Pulmonary artery
   b. Inferior Vena Cava
   c. Aorta
   d. Superior Vena Cava

2. What is the name of the sac that the heart sits in?
   a. Atria
   b. Pericardium
   c. Endocardium
   d. Ventricle

3. What are the three layers of the heart called?
   a. Visceral, Parietal, Membranous
   b. Intima, Media, Adventitia
   c. Fossa ovalis, Foramen ovale, Sinus Venosus
   d. Epicardium, Myocardium, Endocardium

4. The aortic and pulmonic valves are considered what type of valves?
   a. Semilunar valves
   b. Anterior valves
   c. Posterior valves
   d. Atrioventricular valves

5. The blood from the coronary sinus is _____, drains from _____, and drains into the _____.
   a. Unoxygenated; the heart; left ventricle
   b. Unoxygenated; the heart; right atrium
   c. Oxygenated; pulmonary veins; left atrium
   d. Oxygenated; intracardiac shunt; left ventricle

6. Choose the correct pathway (first to last) of the conduction
   a. Purkinje fibers, bundle of His, AV node, SA node
   b. Bundle of HIs, AV node, SA node, Purkinje fibers
   c. SA node, AV node, Purkinje fibers, bundle of His
   d. SA node, AV node, bundle of His, Purkinje fibers

7. On EKG, which wave is produced because of atrial depolarization caused by the SA node?
   a. QRS wave
   b. T wave
   c. P wave
   d. All of the above

8. What duration (timing) of the EKG does diastole occur?
   a. End of T wave to beginning of next QRS
   b. Beginning of P wave to beginning of QRS
   c. Onset QRS to end of T wave
   d. End of QRS to beginning of P wave

9. Which aortic valve leaflets are visualized in the parasternal long axis view (PLAX)?
   a. Left, non cusps
   b. Right, left cusps
   c. Non, right cusps
   d. Right, non, and left cusps

10. Which mitral valve scallops are closest to the LAA appendage?
    a. A3, P3
    b. A1, P1
    c. A3, P1
    d. A2, P2

Vascular Technology

I. MEMORIZATION EXERCISE

1. Write the key words in your notebook or on note cards. Write the words on one side of the notepaper and then write the definitions on the opposite side of the page or on the back of the paper. If using note cards, write the key word on the front and the definition on the back. *This step should be completed before the lab session begins.*

   Memorize the key word definitions silently for 5 minutes, then work with a lab partner and identify the words you still need help with. List the words here. Add additional rows if needed.

II. COMPREHENSION EXERCISE

1. You will need to write in your notebook. First, change each objective into a question.

   Example: "Describe the anatomy of the extracranial vascular system" becomes "What is the anatomy of the extracranial vascular system?"

   Next, write a short answer to the question just created.

   Example: "The anatomy of the extracranial cerebrovascular vessels consists of common carotid arteries, internal carotid arteries, external carotid arteries, and the vertebral arteries."

   Highlight or circle any part of your answers about which you are unsure, and check the answers in your textbook. If you are still unsure of the answers, put a question mark next to the answer(s) for the review session of the lab.

III. APPLICATION OF ANATOMY AND PHYSIOLOGY EXERCISE

1. Label as many major arteries and veins of the head and extremities as you can from the diagrams below. Include each structure's orientation in the body (either vertical, horizontal, vertical oblique, or horizontal oblique). Below your drawing, write two or three summary sentences about the physiology of the vasculature. Ask your lab partner to critique your work. Now check it against the physiology section in the textbook. What did you miss?

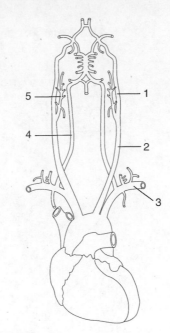

1	_____	4	_____
2	_____	5	_____
3	_____		

Figure 31.1 in the textbook

Physiology: _____

_____

_____

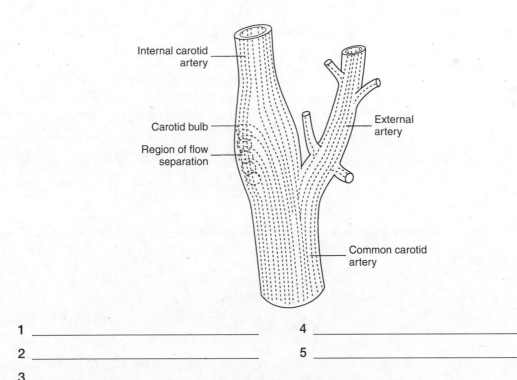

Internal carotid artery

Carotid bulb

Region of flow separation

External artery

Common carotid artery

1	_____	4	_____
2	_____	5	_____
3	_____		

Figure 31.14 in the textbook

Physiology: _____

_____

_____

325

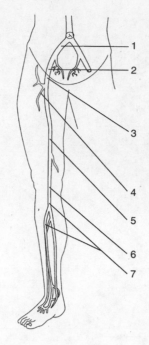

1	_____	5	_____
2	_____	6	_____
3	_____	7	_____
4	_____		

Figure 31.20A in the textbook

Physiology: _____

_____

_____

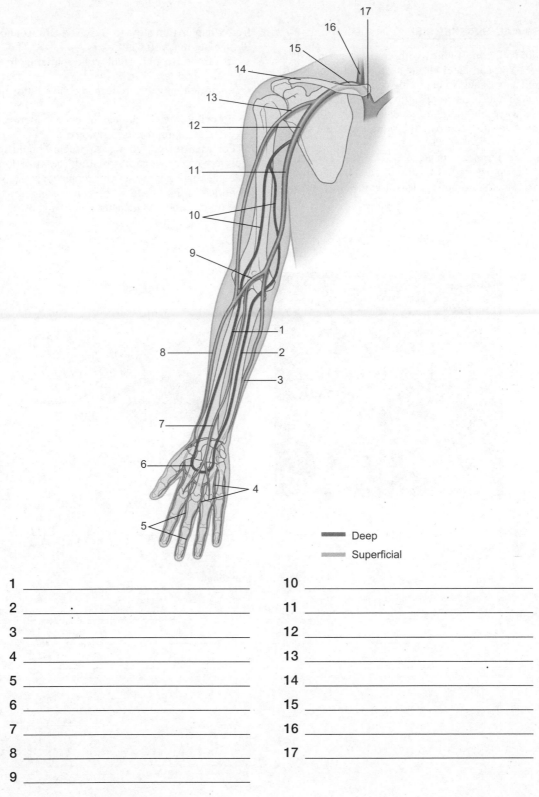

Figure 31.21 in the textbook (From Grant A. and Waugh A. Ross and Wilson Anatomy and Physiology in Health and Illness, 13th ed., Edinburgh, 2018, Elsevier.)

Deep

Superficial

1 _____   10 _____

2 _____   11 _____

3 _____   12 _____

4 _____   13 _____

5 _____   14 _____

6 _____   15 _____

7 _____   16 _____

8 _____   17 _____

9 _____

Physiology: _____

_____

IV. IMAGE ANALYSIS EXERCISE

Work on the following figures with your lab partner. It's your choice! You can label all the sketches at once, then go back and label each image with your lab partner, or label an image and its accompanying sketch at the same time. Either way, the goal is to label correctly all of the sketches and carefully compare the sketch with the sonographic image.

For each sonographic image, write a brief observation that could be "presented" to your instructor, a clinical sonographer, or a sonologist. Please review the section from Chapter 1 on How to Describe Ultrasound Findings. Remember that you want to:

- **differentiate** abnormal echo patterns from normal echo patterns,
- **document** any differences in echo pattern appearance, and
- **describe** any difference in echo pattern appearance using sonographic terminology.

For each image, your assessment should include (1) the view of each major structure (axial or longitudinal; note: these are not the scanning planes) and (2) structures identified in the image with correct sonographic appearance description and measurements if shown.

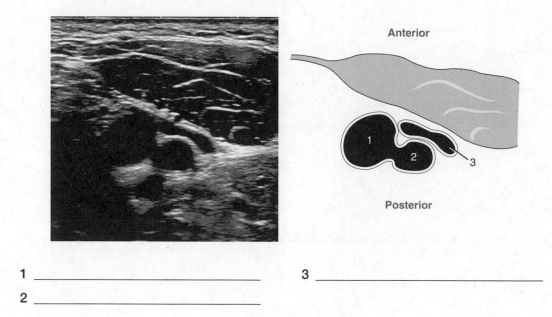

1 _____   3 _____

2 _____

Figure 31.3 in the textbook

Description: _____

_____

_____

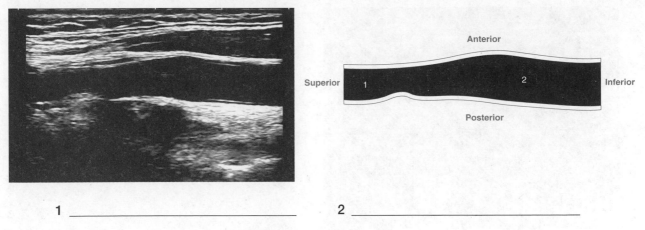

1 _____ 2 _____

Figure 31.7 in the textbook

Description: _____

_____

_____

1 _____ 2 _____

Figure 31.10 in the textbook

Description: _____

_____

_____

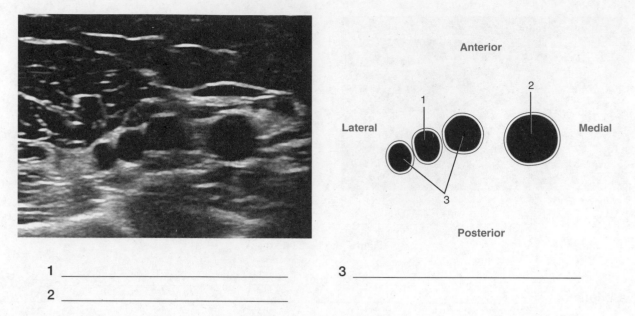

Anterior

Lateral

Medial

1

2

3

Posterior

1 _____   3 _____
2 _____

Figure 31.22 in the textbook

Description: _____

_____

_____

Anterior

Lateral

Medial

1

2

3

Posterior

1 _____   3 _____
2 _____

Figure 31.29 in the textbook

Description: _____

_____

Chapter **31** **Vascular Technology**

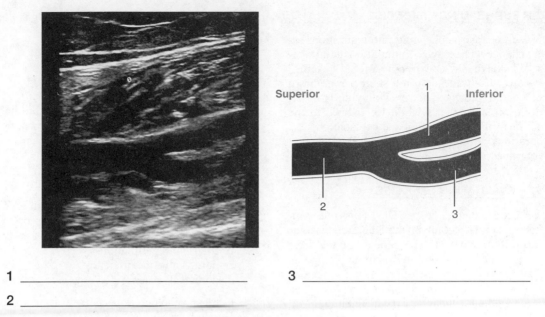

Superior   Inferior

1 _____   3 _____

2 _____

Figure 31.30 in the textbook

Description: _____

_____

_____

V. CHAPTER SUBHEADINGS EXERCISE

1. Convert each chapter subheading into a question; for example, change "The Lower Extremity Arterial System" to "What is the lower extremity arterial system?" Briefly answer each question in a short paragraph in your notebook. Exchange answers with your lab partner and check each other's work. Refer back to the textbook for further information and explanation.
2. What questions do you still have about the chapter? Write your questions in your notebook.

VI. CHAPTER EVALUATION EXERCISE

Use a fresh sheet of notebook paper. Based on your work with the chapter and its accompanying laboratory assignments, identify three concepts you believe are the most important. You may draw from any of the assignments you've already completed in the previous pages, including learning objectives, anatomy and physiology, images, or chapter subheadings. Include a detailed rationale in your answers.

Answer the questions below. Refer to page 372 for the answers.

1. The intracranial branch of the ICA is
   a. superficial temporal.
   b. ophthalmic.
   c. facial.
   d. maxillary.

2. The vertebral artery is a branch of the
   a. aortic arch.
   b. common carotid artery.
   c. subclavian artery.
   d. innominate artery.

3. The percentage of the population that have an intact Circle of Willis is
   a. 90%.
   b. 55%.
   c. > 50%.
   d. < 50%.

4. Which imaging modality is best at evaluating the vessel walls for plaque formation?
   a. Gray-scale imaging
   b. Color Doppler
   c. Power Doppler
   d. Spectral Doppler

5. Which imaging modality supplies physiologic information of blood flow in a vessel?
   a. Gray-scale imaging
   b. Color Doppler
   c. Power Doppler
   d. Spectral Doppler

6. The spectral Doppler waveforms from an extracranial imaging exam are directly impacted by
   a. cardiac status and output.
   b. the temperature of the room.
   c. patient fasting.
   d. patient sleeping during exam.

7. The spectral Doppler waveform with a double systolic peak signifies that a patient has
   a. cardiomyopathy.
   b. tricuspid regurgitation.
   c. aortic valve insufficiency.
   d. aortic valve stenosis.

8. Cardiac pathology impacts the carotid vessel spectral Doppler waveforms
   a. intermittently.
   b. bilaterally.
   c. have no impact on the carotid vessel waveforms.
   d. unilaterally.

9. A high resistive spectral Doppler waveform is associated with a normal
   a. ICA.
   b. vertebral.
   c. CCA.
   d. ECA.

10. The change in vessel diameter from the CCA to the bulb creates a normal flow pattern called
    a. low resistance.
    b. boundary layer separation.
    c. high resistance.
    d. turbulence.

3D/4D/5D Sonography

I. MEMORIZATION EXERCISE

1. Write the key words in your notebook or on note cards. Write the words on one side of the notepaper and then write the definitions on the opposite side of the page or on the back of the paper. If using note cards, write the key word on the front and the definition on the back. *This step should be completed before the lab session begins.*

   Memorize the key word definitions silently for 5 minutes, then work with a lab partner and identify the words you still need help with. List the words here. Add additional rows if needed.

II. COMPREHENSION EXERCISE

1. Work with a lab partner to complete this exercise. You will need to write in your notebook. First, change each objective into a question.

   Example: "Define three-dimensional (3D) sonography" becomes "What is three-dimensional (3D) sonography?"

2. Next, write a short answer to the question just created.

   Example: "Three-dimensional sonography is an evolving technology that allows images to be viewed in three dimensions instead of the traditional two-dimensional viewing. It can be divided into three steps: volume acquisition, multiplanar display, and three-dimensional rendering. Real-time three-dimensional sonography is sometimes called four-dimensional sonography, where the fourth dimension is time."

3. Highlight or circle any part of your answers about which you are unsure, and check the answers in your textbook. If you are still unsure of the answers, put a question mark next to the answer(s) for the review session of the lab.

III. APPLICATION OF ANATOMY AND PHYSIOLOGY EXERCISE

1. Using a piece of paper or clay, create a three-dimensional structure of the kidney. Label the kidney; include the structure's orientation in the body (either vertical, horizontal, vertical oblixque, or horizontal oblique). Ask your lab partner to critique your work. What did you miss?

   Check your model using the three-dimensional images in your textbook and complete any structures missing from your model.

2. Write two or three summary sentences about three-dimensional imaging. Ask your lab partner to check your work. What else can you add to your description?

IV. IMAGE ANALYSIS EXERCISE

Work on the following figures with a lab partner, a group or independently. The goal is to label correctly all of the sketches and carefully compare the sketch with the sonographic image.

For each sonographic image, write a brief observation that could be "presented" to your instructor, a clinical sonographer, or a sonologist. Please review the section from Chapter 1 on How to Describe Ultrasound Findings. Remember that you want to:

- **differentiate** abnormal echo patterns from normal echo patterns,
- **document** any differences in echo pattern appearance, and
- **describe** any difference in echo pattern appearance using sonographic terminology.

For each image, your assessment should include (1) the view of each major structure (axial or longitudinal) and (2) structures identified in the image with correct sonographic appearance description and measurements if shown.

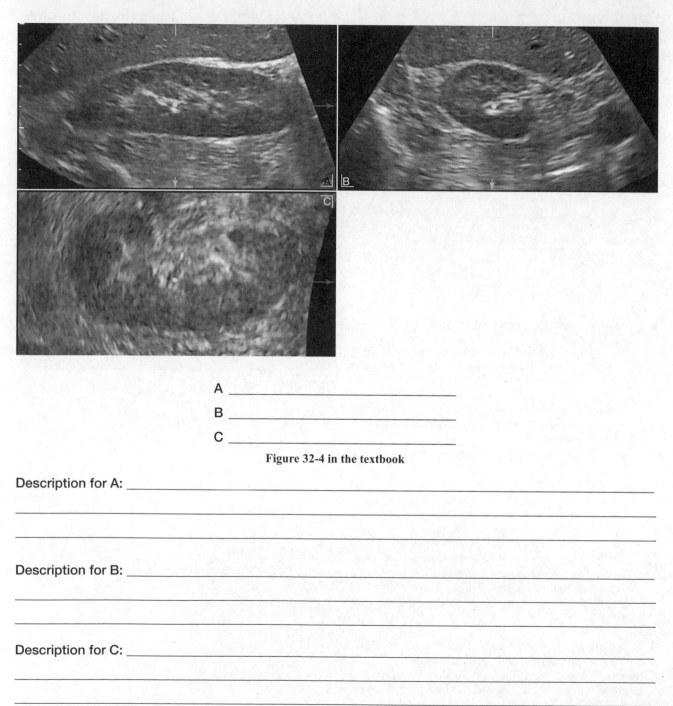

A _____

B _____

C _____

Figure 32-4 in the textbook

Description for A: _____

_____

_____

Description for B: _____

_____

_____

Description for C: _____

_____

_____

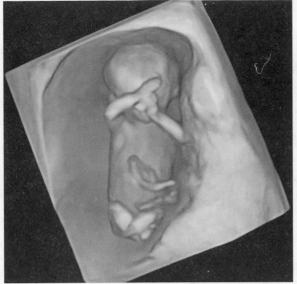

1 _____

Figure 32-10 in the textbook

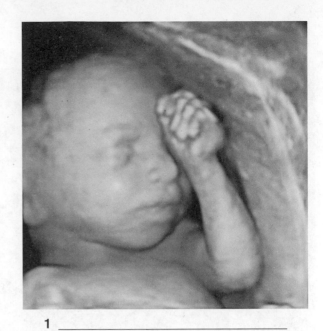

1 _____

Figure 32-20 in the textbook

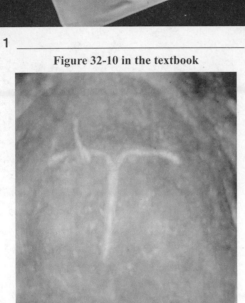

1 _____

Figure 32-21 in the textbook

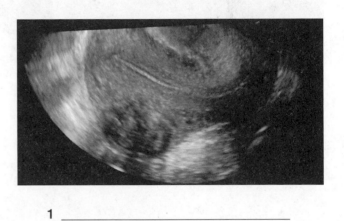

1 _____

Figure 32-25 in the textbook

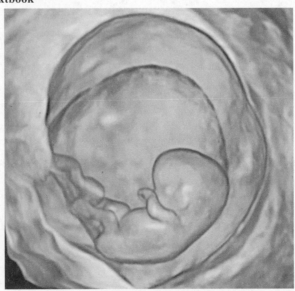

1 _____

Figure 32-26 in the textbook

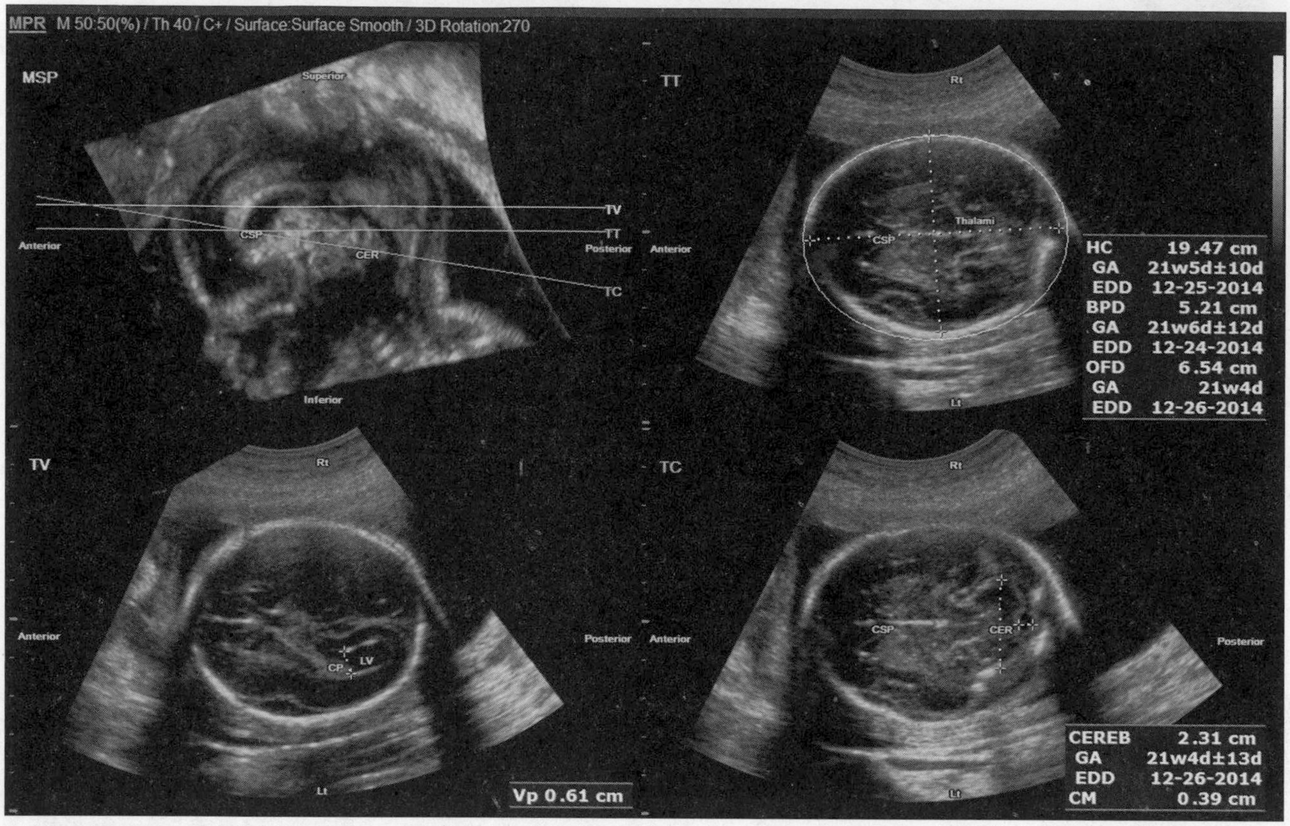

Figure 32-42B in the textbook

A _____

B _____

C _____

3D _____

Description for A: _____

_____

_____

Description for B: _____

_____

_____

Description for C: _____

_____

_____

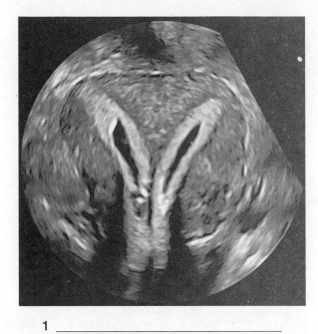

1 _____

Figure 32-29 in the textbook

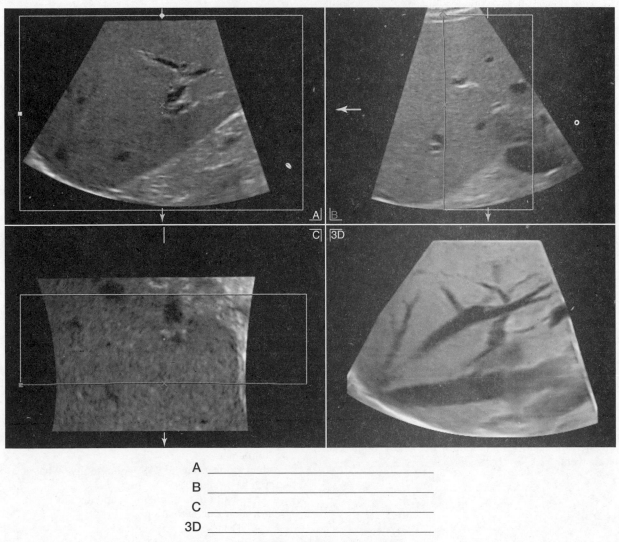

A _____
B _____
C _____
3D _____

Figure 32-30 in the textbook

Chapter **32** **3D/4D/5D Sonography**

Description for A: _____

_____

_____

Description for B: _____

_____

_____

Description for C: _____

_____

_____

V. CHAPTER SUBHEADINGS EXERCISE

1. Convert each chapter subheading into a question; for example, change "Sonographic Applications" to "What are the sonographic applications of 3D/4D sonography?" Briefly answer each question in a short paragraph in your notebook. Exchange answers with your lab partner and check each other's work. Refer back to the textbook for further information and explanation

2. What questions do you still have about the chapter? Write your questions in your notebook.

VI. CHAPTER EVALUATION EXERCISE

Use a fresh sheet of notebook paper. Based on your work with the chapter and its accompanying laboratory assignments, identify three concepts you believe are the most important. You may draw from any of the assignments you've already completed in the previous pages, including learning objectives, anatomy and physiology, images, or chapter subheadings. Include a detailed rationale in your answers.

Answer the questions below. Refer to page 372 for the answers.

Multiple Choice

1. Congenital uterine malformations are best visualized in which imaging plane?
   a. Axial
   b. Sagittal
   c. Coronal
   d. Longitudinal
2. 5D sonography
   a. is also known as real-time 3D.
   b. is not approved for diagnostic use in the United States.
   c. is performed using manual, timed, frame-averaging techniques.
   d. represents the automated quantification from 3D or 4D volume datasets.
3. What is the axis dot referring to in volume imaging?
   a. The reference plane for the volume dataset.
   b. The reference location of the volume dataset.
   c. The point at the intersection of the orthogonal planes in a multiplanar display.
   d. The point at the very center of the coronal plane in a multiplanar display.
4. Thick slice volume imaging is useful to
   a. enhance visualization of the fetal ribs in the C-plane.
   b. display a single fetal cardiac cycle in motion.
   c. quickly measure anatomy within the volume dataset.
   d. label normal and abnormal anatomy within the volume dataset.
5. When performing 3D/4D sonography, what are the three basic steps?
   a. Acquisition, manipulation, and display
   b. X-, Y-, Z-axis rotation
   c. A-, B-, C-plane acquisition
   d. Orthogonal, axial and coronal display

6. What should the sonographer do to demonstrate the shadowing from the gallstones simultaneously in all three orthogonal planes?

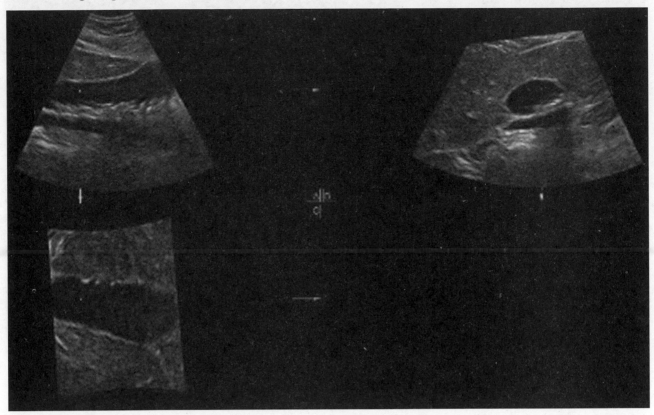

a. Prior to the 3D volume acquisition, increase the volume angle.
b. Prior to the 3D volume acquisition, increase the volume quality.
c. Move the axis dot to be positioned in the gallstones' shadow.
d. Use the "Z-technique" to align the volume dataset.

7. This is a volume rendering of a thyroid. The arrow in the rendered image is pointing to the

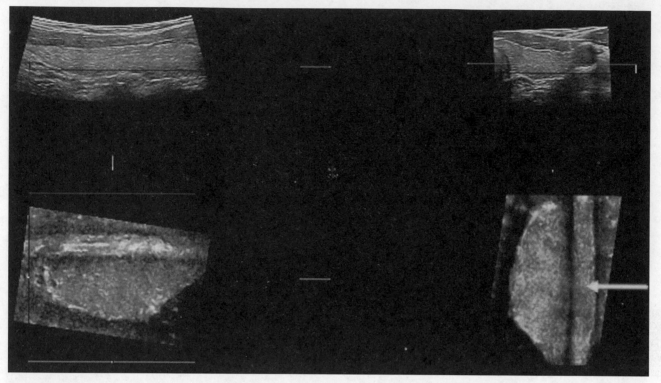

a. carotid artery.
b. thyroid lobe.
c. isthmus.
d. tongue.

8. The image below is an example of using minimum render mode to demonstrate liver vasculature. What is the arrow pointing to?

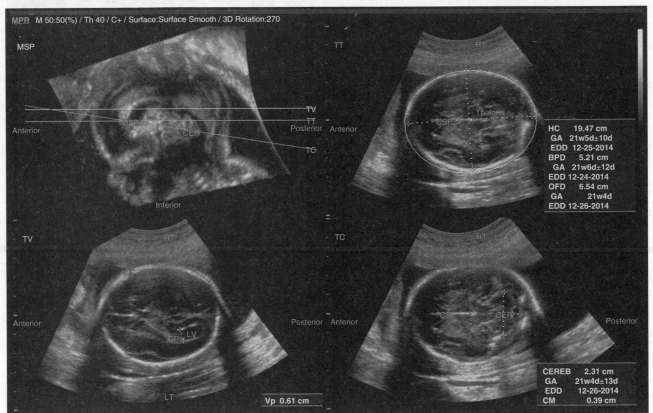

a. Kidney cyst
b. Portal vein
c. Left hepatic vein
d. Gallbladder

9. When using 3D sonography in breast imaging, what is the most useful imaging plane for diagnosis?
a. Axial
b. Coronal
c. Sagittal
d. Oblique

10. True/False: 3D, 4D, and 5D technologies can generate fetal aortic and ductal arch images from a 4-chamber heart imaging plane.
a. True
b. False

Interventional and Intraoperative Ultrasound 33

I. MEMORIZATION EXERCISE

1. Write the key words in your notebook or on note cards. Write the words on one side of the notepaper and then write the definitions on the opposite side of the page or on the back of the paper. If using note cards, write the key word on the front and the definition on the back. *This step should be completed before the lab session begins.*

   Memorize the key word definitions silently for 5 minutes, then work with a lab partner and identify the words you still need help with. List the words here. Add additional rows if needed.

II. COMPREHENSION EXERCISE

1. Work with a lab partner to complete this exercise. You will need to write in your notebook. First, change the objective into a question.

   Example: "Understand ultrasound-assisted interventional and intraoperative procedures" becomes "What are ultrasound-assisted interventional and intraoperative procedures?"

   Next, write a short answer to the question just created.

   Example: "Interventional sonography is the use of sonographic procedures to assist the physician in completing an invasive procedure, such as an endoscopic examination of the pancreas."

Highlight or circle any part of your answers about which you are unsure, and check the answers in your textbook. If you are still unsure of the answers, put a question mark next to the answer(s) for the review session of the lab.

III. APPLICATION OF ANATOMY AND PHYSIOLOGY EXERCISE

1. Write two or three summary sentences about interventional sonographic imaging and two or three summary sentences about intraoperative sonographic imaging. Include in your description the similarities and differences in procedures and applicable use. Ask your lab partner to check your work. What else can you add to your description?

IV. IMAGE ANALYSIS EXERCISE

Work on the following figures with your lab partner. It's your choice! You can label all the sketches at once, then go back and label each image with your lab partner, or label an image and its accompanying sketch at the same time. Either way, the goal is to label correctly all of the sketches and carefully compare the sketch with the sonographic image.

For each sonographic image, write a brief observation that could be "presented" to your instructor, a clinical sonographer, or a sonologist. Please review the section from Chapter 1 on How to Describe Ultrasound Findings. Remember that you want to:

- **differentiate** abnormal echo patterns from normal echo patterns,
- **document** any differences in echo pattern appearance, and
- **describe** any difference in echo pattern appearance using sonographic terminology.

For each image, your assessment should include (1) the view of each major structure (axial or longitudinal; note: these are not the scanning planes) and (2) structures identified in the image with correct sonographic appearance description and measurements if shown.

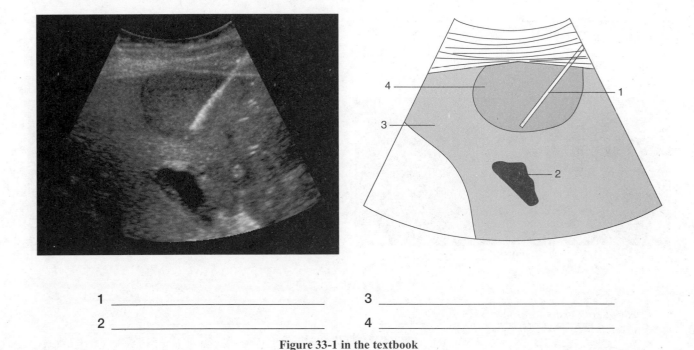

1 _____   3 _____

2 _____   4 _____

Figure 33-1 in the textbook

Description: _____
_____
_____

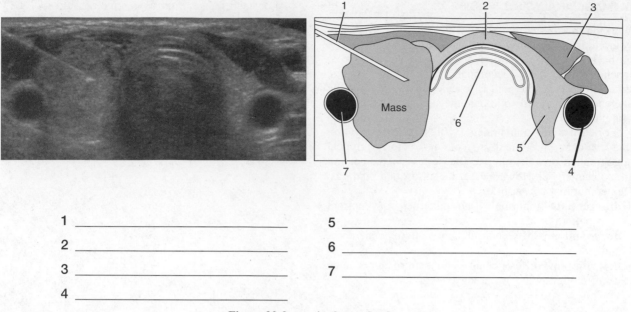

1	_____	5	_____
2	_____	6	_____
3	_____	7	_____
4	_____		

Figure 33-2, top, in the textbook

Description: _____

_____

_____

| 1 | _____ | 3 | _____ |
| 2 | _____ | 4 | _____ |

Figure 33-3 in the textbook

Description: _____

_____

_____

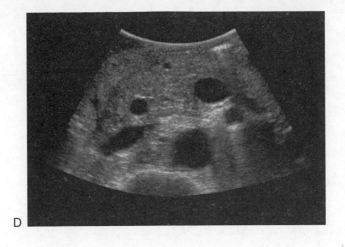

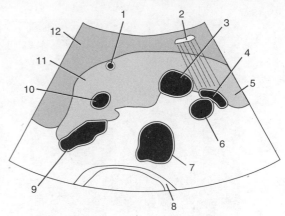

1	_____	7	_____
2	_____	8	_____
3	_____	9	_____
4	_____	10	_____
5	_____	11	_____
6	_____	12	_____

Figure 33.5D in the textbook

Description: _____

_____

_____

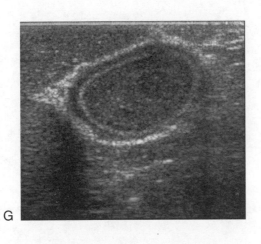

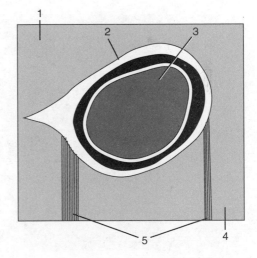

1	_____	4	_____
2	_____	5	_____
3	_____		

Figure 33.5G in the textbook

Description: _____

_____

_____

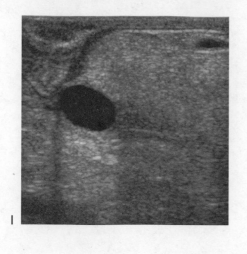
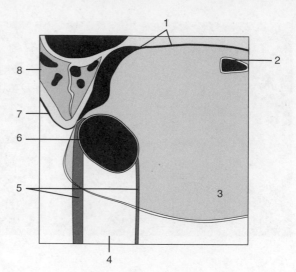

1	_____	5	_____
2	_____	6	_____
3	_____	7	_____
4	_____		

Figure 33.5I in the textbook

Description: _____

_____

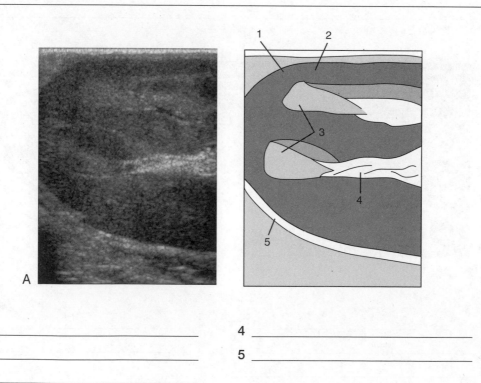

1	_____	4	_____
2	_____	5	_____
3	_____		

Figure 33-6A in the textbook

Description: _____

_____

346

Chapter **33** Interventional and Intraoperative Ultrasound

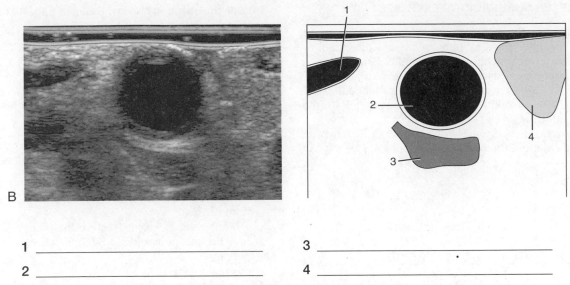

B

1 _____   3 _____

2 _____   4 _____

Figure 33-7B in the textbook

V. CHAPTER SUBHEADINGS EXERCISE

1. Convert each chapter subheading into a question; for example, change "Intraoperative Ultrasound" to "What is intraoperative ultrasound?" Briefly answer each question in a short paragraph in your notebook.

   Exchange answers with your lab partner and check each other's work. Refer back to the textbook for further information and explanation.

2. What questions do you still have about the chapter? Write your questions in your notebook.

VI. CHAPTER EVALUATION EXERCISE

Use a fresh sheet of notebook paper. Based on your work with the chapter and its accompanying laboratory assignments, identify three concepts you believe are the most important. You may draw from any of the assignments you've already completed in the previous pages, including learning objectives, anatomy and physiology, images, or chapter subheadings. Include a detailed rationale in your answers.

Answer the questions below. Refer to page 373 for the answers.

Multiple Choice

1. Which of the following is an advantage of interventional and intraoperative procedures?
   a. Nonvisualization of needle placement
   b. Needle or tube tracking
   c. Need for ionizing radiation
   d. Limited to biopsies
2. Intraoperative ultrasound is NOT limited by
   a. air.
   b. fluid.
   c. the need for ionizing radiation.
   d. sterile fields.
3. A biopsy site is scanned before the biopsy to determine the best point of entry with the shortest distance and the
   a. smallest angle.
   b. largest angle.
   c. smallest track.
   d. clearest sterile field.
4. During an ultrasound-guided aspiration,
   a. chorionic villus sampling is performed.
   b. any change in the shape or size of a fluid-filled structure can be visualized.
   c. the transducer is endoluminal.
   d. a laparoscopic transducer is always used.
5. Ultrasound is used during _____ to determine accurate needle placement for tissue sampling.
   a. percutaneous aspiration
   b. percutaneous cholangiogram
   c. cyst aspiration
   d. percutaneous biopsies

True/False

6. Percutaneous aspirations obtain tissue samples by applying suction through a needle attached to a syringe. ___

7. Ultrasound-guided biopsies use ultrasound to determine accurate needle placement for fluid suction. ___

8. An option for a sterile transducer sheath during interventional ultrasound is an alcohol bath. ___

9. Ultrasound-guided aspirations assist needle placement for small organ or stone extraction. ___

10. Chorionic villus sampling is considered a percutaneous biopsy procedure. ___

34 Musculoskeletal Sonography

I. MEMORIZATION EXERCISE

1. Write the key words in your notebook or on note cards. Write the words on one side of the notepaper and then write the definitions on the opposite side of the page or on the back of the paper. If using note cards, write the key word on the front and the definition on the back. *This step should be completed before the lab session begins.*

   Memorize the key word definitions silently for 5 minutes, then work with a lab partner and identify the words you still need help with. List the words here. Add additional rows if needed.

II. COMPREHENSION EXERCISE

1. Work with a lab partner to complete this exercise. You will need to write in your notebook. First, change each objective into a question.

   Example: "Explain the function of the musculoskeletal system" becomes "What is the function of the musculoskeletal system?"

   Next, write a short answer to the question just created. You can divide the answer into parts.

   Example: "The musculoskeletal system is comprised of muscles, tendons, ligaments, cartilage, and nerves. Muscles facilitate movement, tendons attach muscles to bones, ligaments connect bones to bones, cartilage assists with smooth movement in the joints, and nerves transmit impulses to the brain, spinal cord (the central nervous system)."

   Highlight or circle any part of your answers about which you are unsure, and check the answers in your textbook. If you are still unsure of the answers, put a question mark next to the answer(s) for the review session of the lab.

1. Label the diagrams below. Ask your lab partner to critique your work. What did you miss? Check your labeling using Figures 34-6A, 34-6B and 34-14 in your textbook and complete any missing anatomical structures.

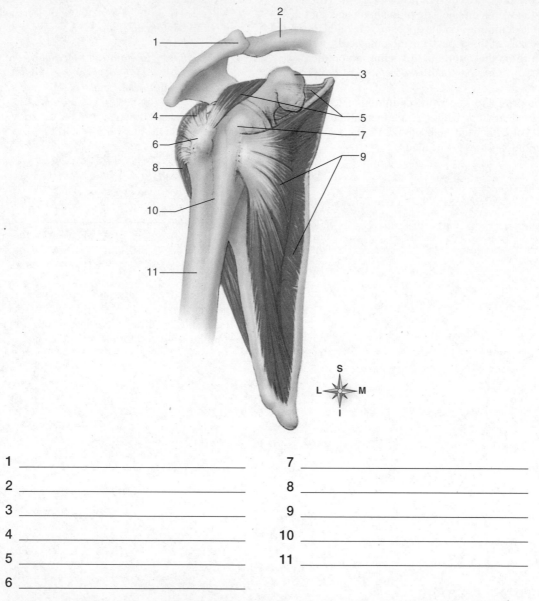

1 _____	7 _____
2 _____	8 _____
3 _____	9 _____
4 _____	10 _____
5 _____	11 _____
6 _____	

Figure 34-6A in the textbook From Patton K.T., Thibodeau G.A. Anthony's Textbook of Anatomy & Physiology, 21st ed, St. Louis, 2019, Elsevier.

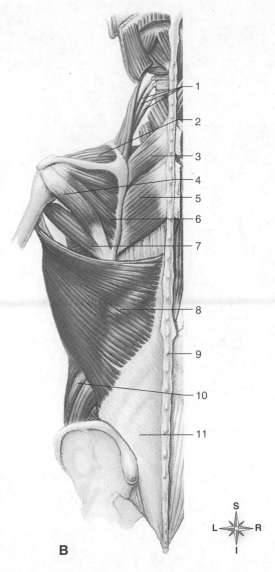

1 _____

2 _____

3 _____

4 _____

5 _____

6 _____

7 _____

8 _____

9 _____

10 _____

11 _____

B

Figure 34-6B in the textbook From Patton K.T., Thibodeau G.A. Anthony's Textbook of Anatomy & Physiology, 21st ed, St. Louis, 2019, Elsevier.

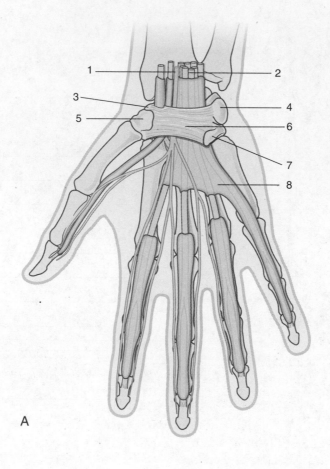

A

1 _____   5 _____

2 _____   6 _____

3 _____   7 _____

4 _____   8 _____

Figure 34-14A in the textbook From Grant A. and Waugh A. Ross & Wilson Anatomy and Physiology in Health and Illness, 13th ed, Edinburgh, 2018, Elsevier.

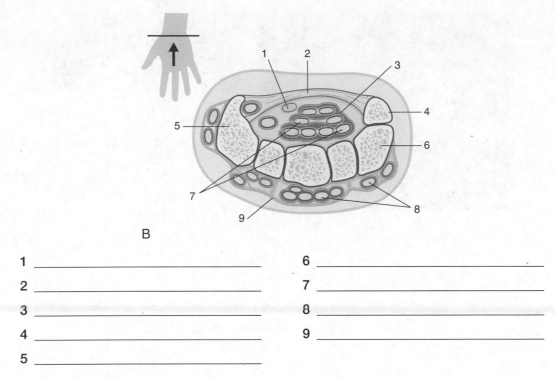

B

1	_____	6	_____
2	_____	7	_____
3	_____	8	_____
4	_____	9	_____
5	_____		

Figure 34-14B in the textbook From Grant A. and Waugh A. Ross & Wilson Anatomy and Physiology in Health and Illness, 13th ed, Edinburgh, 2018, Elsevier.

2. Write two or three summary sentences about the anatomy of the rotator cuff. Ask your lab partner to check your work. Now check your work against the physiology section in the textbook. What else can you add to your description?

_____

_____

_____

3. Write two or three summary sentences about the anatomy of the carpal tunnel. Ask your lab partner to check your work. Now check your work against the physiology section in the textbook. What else can you add to your description?

_____

_____

_____

IV. IMAGE ANALYSIS EXERCISE

Work on the following figures with your lab partner. It's your choice! You can label all the sketches at once, then go back and label each image with your lab partner, or label an image and its accompanying sketch at the same time. Either way, the goal is to label correctly all of the sketches and carefully compare the sketch with the sonographic image.

For each sonographic image, write a brief observation that could be "presented" to your instructor, a clinical sonographer, or a sonologist. Please review the section from Chapter 1 on How to Describe Ultrasound Findings. Remember that you want to:

- **differentiate** abnormal echo patterns from normal echo patterns,
- **document** any differences in echo pattern appearance, and
- **describe** any difference in echo pattern appearance using sonographic terminology.

For each image, your assessment should include (1) the view of each major structure (axial or longitudinal; note: these are not the scanning planes) and (2) structures identified in the image with correct sonographic appearance description and measurements if shown.

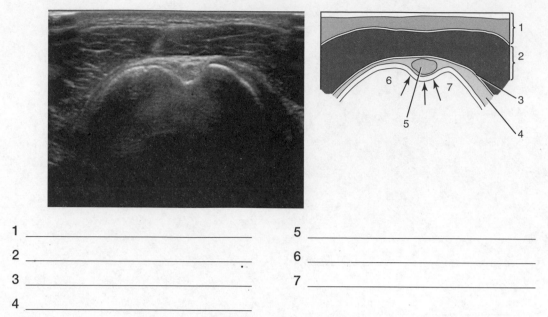

1	_____	5	_____
2	_____	6	_____
3	_____	7	_____
4	_____		

Figure 34-7 in the textbook

Description:

_____

_____

_____

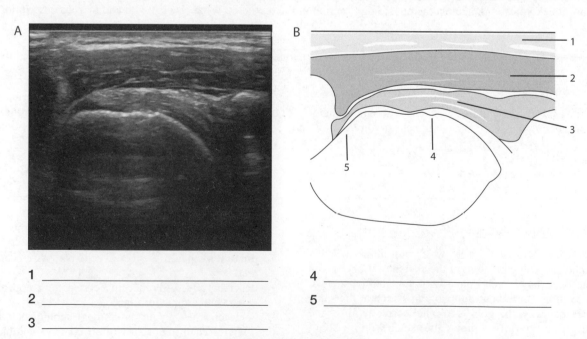

1	_____	4	_____
2	_____	5	_____
3	_____		

Figure 34-8 in the textbook

Description:

_____

_____

_____

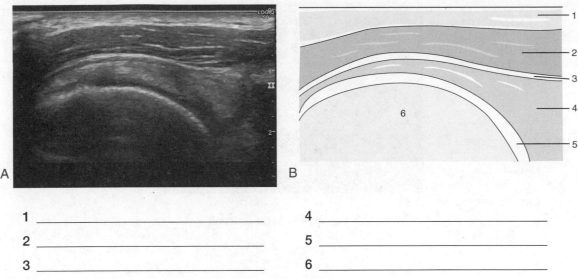

A

B

1 _____   4 _____
2 _____   5 _____
3 _____   6 _____

Figure 34-10 in the textbook

Description:

_____
_____
_____

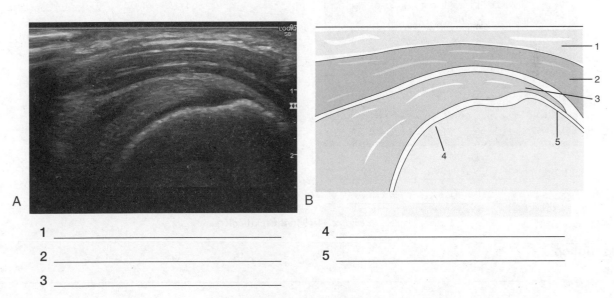

A

B

1 _____   4 _____
2 _____   5 _____
3 _____

Figure 34-11 in the textbook

Description:

_____
_____
_____

Chapter **34** **Musculoskeletal Sonography**

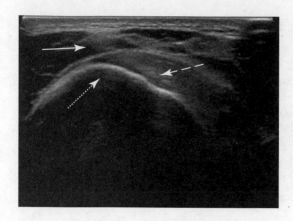

Figure 34-12 in the textbook

Description:

_____

_____

_____

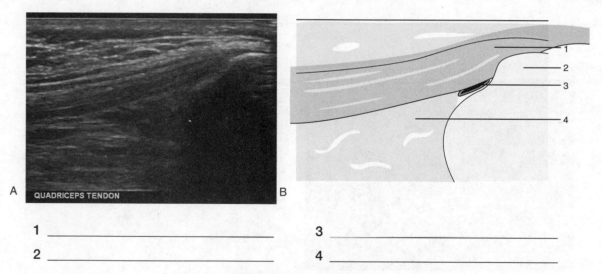

A   QUADRICEPS TENDON   B

1 _____   3 _____

2 _____   4 _____

Figure 34-19 in the textbook

Description:

_____

_____

_____

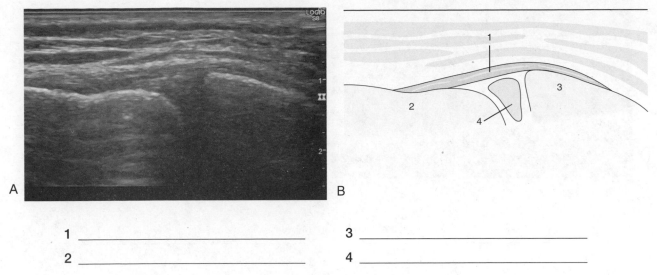

1 _____   3 _____
2 _____   4 _____

Figure 34-21 in the textbook

Description:

_____

_____

_____

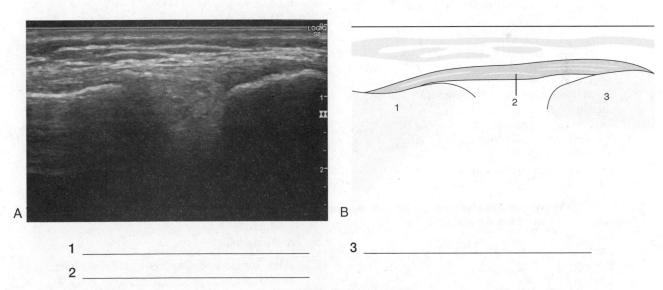

1 _____   3 _____
2 _____

Figure 34-22 in the textbook

Description:

_____

_____

_____

Chapter **34** **Musculoskeletal Sonography**

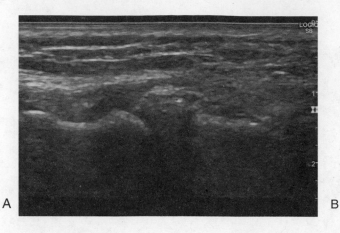

A

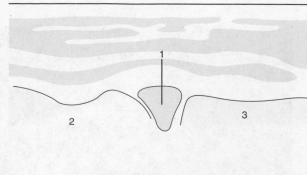

B

1 _____   3 _____

2 _____

Figure 34-23 in the textbook

Description:

_____

_____

_____

V. CHAPTER EVALUATION EXERCISE

Answer the question below. Refer to page 373 for the answers.

Multiple Choice

1. At what location are most tears of the achilles tendon?
   a. Distal tendon at the attachment to the soleus muscle
   b. Proximal attachment to the calcaneus bone
   c. 2–6 cm proximal to the attachment to the calcaneus bone
   d. 2–6 cm distal to the attachment to the soleus muscle

2. What is the maximum measurement of the achilles tendon considered within normal limits?
   a. 3 cm
   b. 4 cm
   c. 5 cm
   d. 6 cm

3. The achilles tendon attaches to what bone?
   a. Calcaneus
   b. Humeral head
   c. Radius
   d. Tibia

4. What material covers the ends of many long bones to promote movement and cushion the space between the bones?
   a. Bursa
   b. Hyaline cartilage
   c. Menisci
   d. Enthesis

5. What part of the musculoskeletal system connects bones to muscles?
   a. Tendons
   b. Ligaments
   c. Cartilage
   d. Bursa

6. What is the largest synovial joint in the body?
   a. Knee joint
   b. Shoulder joint
   c. Hip joint
   d. Ankle joint

7. What are the bony landmarks for the medial collateral ligament?
   a. Femur and fibula
   b. Femur and tibia
   c. Femur and patella
   d. Tibia and fibula

8. What dynamic movement might help to distinguish the median nerve from the adjacent tendons?
   a. Flexion of the wrist showing movement of the tendons
   b. Flexion of four of the fingers showing movement of the tendons
   c. Flexion of the wrist showing movement of the nerve
   d. Flexion of four of the fingers showing movement of the nerve

9. What is the tough fibrocartilage on the lateral and medial knee that helps provide stabilization of the knee joint?

   a. Hyaline cartilage
   b. Bursae
   c. Menisci
   d. Lateral and medial collateral ligaments

10. Which statement is true regarding bursae?
    a. Bursae always contain fluid that is perceivable by ultrasound.
    b. Bursae never contain fluid that is perceivable by ultrasound.
    c. If the bursae contain any amount of fluid it is an abnormal finding.
    d. Bursae may naturally contain visible fluid; abnormal findings are based on the amount of fluid.

35 Pediatric Sonography

I. MEMORIZATION EXERCISE

1. Write the key words in your notebook or on note cards. Write the words on one side of the notepaper and then write the definitions on the opposite side of the page or on the back of the paper. If using note cards, write the key word on the front and the definition on the back. *This step should be completed before the lab session begins.*

   Memorize the key word definitions silently for 5 minutes, then work with a lab partner and identify the words you still need help with. List the words here. Add additional rows if needed.

II. COMPREHENSION EXERCISE

1. Work with a lab partner to complete this exercise. You will need to write in your notebook. First, change each objective into a question.

   Example: "List normal variants and congenital anomalies of organs in the pediatric patient" becomes *"What are normal variants and congenital anomalies of the liver?"*

   Next, write a short answer to the question just created.

   Example: "Normal variants and congenital anomalies of the liver include Riedel's lobe, situs inversus and congenital absence of the left lobe."

You should be able to write a similar question and answers for each pediatric organ and system given in this chapter.

Highlight or circle any part of your answers about which you are unsure, and check the answers in your textbook. If you are still unsure of the answers, put a question mark next to the answer(s) for the review session of the lab.

III. APPLICATION OF ANATOMY AND PHYSIOLOGY EXERCISE

1. In your notebook, draw the right and left adrenal glands and as much proximal anatomy as you can from memory. Refer to Figures 35-7A and 35-7B to check your drawings.

2. Label the normal hip joint as viewed in the coronal image plane. Include each structure's orientation in the body (either vertical, horizontal, vertical oblique, or horizontal oblique). Ask your lab partner to critique your work. What did you miss? Check your drawing using Figure 35-17 in your textbook and complete any missing structures from your drawing.

3. Below your drawing, write two or three summary sentences of the physiology of the pediatric hip joint. Ask your lab partner to check your work. Now check your work against the sonographic appearance section on the hip in the textbook. What else can you add to your description?

IV. IMAGE ANALYSIS EXERCISE

Work on the following figures with your lab partner. Its your choice! You can label all the sketches at once, then go back and label each image with your lab partner, or label an image and its accompanying sketch at the same time. Either way, the goal is to label correctly all of the sketches and carefully compare the sketch with the sonographic image.

For each sonographic image, write a brief observation that could be presented to your instructor, a clinical sonographer, or a sonologist. Please review the section from Chapter 1 on How to Describe Ultrasound Findings. Remember that you want to:

- **differentiate** abnormal echo patterns from normal echo patterns,
- **document** any differences in echo pattern appearance, and
- **describe** any difference in echo pattern appearance using sonographic terminology.

For each image, your assessment should include (1) the view of each major structure (axial or longitudinal; note: these are not the scanning planes) and (2) structures identified in the image with correct sonographic appearance description and measurements if shown.

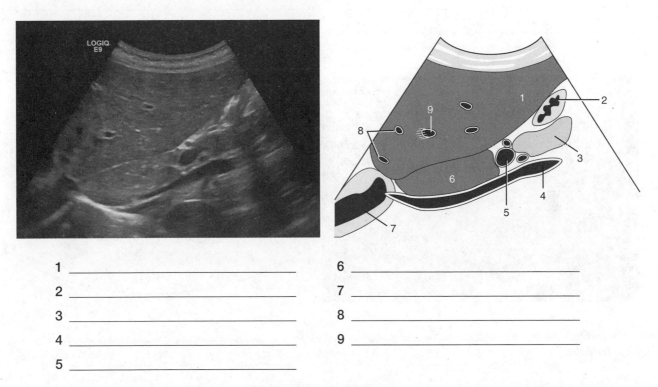

1 _____	6 _____
2 _____	7 _____
3 _____	8 _____
4 _____	9 _____
5 _____	

Figure 35-1 in the textbook

Description:

_____

_____

_____

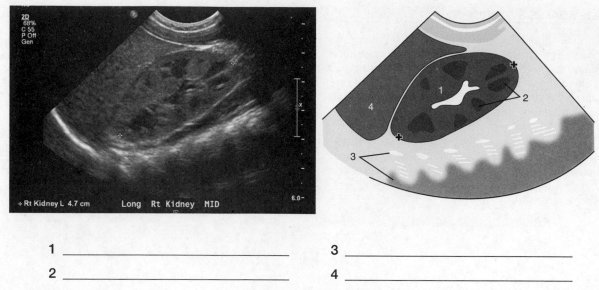

1 _____   3 _____
2 _____   4 _____

Figure 35-2 in the textbook

Description:

_____

_____

_____

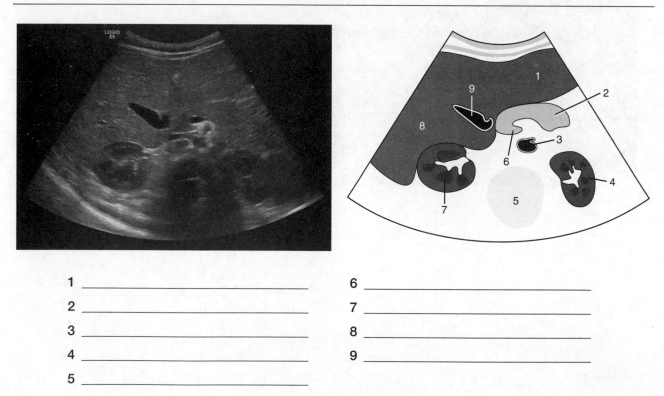

1 _____   6 _____
2 _____   7 _____
3 _____   8 _____
4 _____   9 _____
5 _____

Figure 35-4 in the textbook

Description:

_____

_____

_____

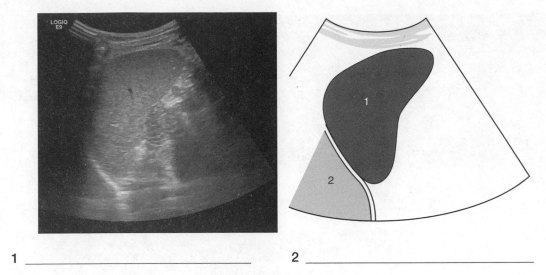

1 _____   2 _____

Figure 35-8 in the textbook

Description:

_____
_____
_____
_____

1 _____   4 _____

2 _____   5 _____

3 _____   6 _____

Figure 35-9 in the textbook

Description:

_____
_____
_____

363

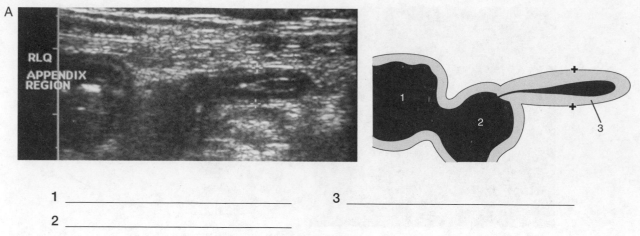

A

RLQ
APPENDIX
REGION

1 _____   3 _____
2 _____

Figure 35-11A in the textbook

Description:

_____

_____

_____

Long Uterus RT

5.0—

1 _____   4 _____
2 _____   5 _____
3 _____   6 _____

Figure 35-12 in the textbook

Description:

_____

_____

_____

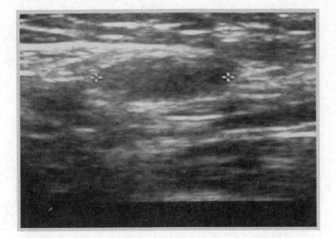

1 _____

Figure 35-14 in the textbook

Description:

_____

_____

_____

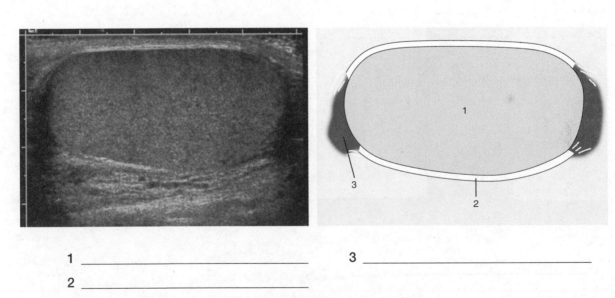

1 _____   3 _____

2 _____

Figure 35-15 in the textbook

Description:

_____

_____

_____

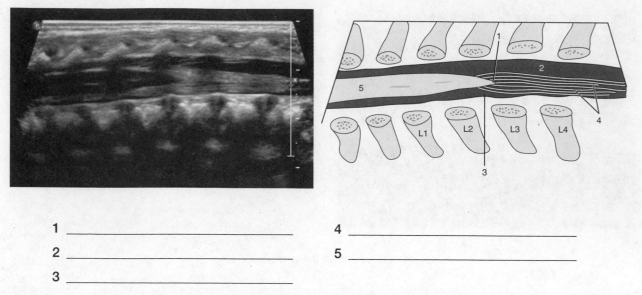

1 _____   4 _____

2 _____   5 _____

3 _____

Figure 35-16 in the textbook

Description:

_____

_____

_____

V. CHAPTER SUBHEADINGS EXERCISE

1. Convert each chapter subheading related to a particular organ into a question; for example, for a question section, write "What are the sonographic applications of the pediatric liver?" Write the answer to each question in a short paragraph in your notebook. Exchange answers with your lab partner and check each other's work. Refer back to the textbook for further information and explanation.

2. What questions do you still have about the chapter? Write your questions in your notebook.

VI CHAPTER EVALUATION EXERCISE

Use a fresh sheet of notebook paper. Based on your work with the chapter and its accompanying laboratory assignments, identify three concepts you believe are the most important. You may draw from any of the assignments you have already completed in the previous pages, including learning objectives, anatomy and physiology, images, or chapter subheadings. Include a detailed rationale in your answers.

Answer the questions below. Refer to page 373 for the answers.

Multiple Choice

1. In a normal spinal ultrasound, between which vertebrae should the tip of the conus end?
   a. L3–L4
   b. T12–L1
   c. L1–L2
   d. S1–S2

2. In which organ can the Riedel lobe, an anatomic variant, be seen?
   a. Spleen
   b. Liver
   c. Gallbladder
   d. Stomach

3. Which structure is often identified on ultrasound connecting breast tissue to the skin?
   a. Areola
   b. Cooper's ligaments
   c. Fibromuscular papilla
   d. Fat lobules

4. What is polythelia?
   a. An accessory nipple
   b. Multiple testicles
   c. An accessory bile duct
   d. An accessory spleen

5. What is the central echo complex in spinal ultrasound?
   a. Conus medullaris
   b. Center of the cord
   c. Vertebral body
   d. Filum terminale

6. Which is the recommended age range to perform hip ultrasound for the evaluation of development dysplasia of the hip?
   a. 2–4 weeks
   b. 4–6 weeks
   c. 6–8 weeks
   d. 8–10 weeks

7. Which of the following is one of the most common inherited pancreatic diseases of childhood?
   a. Caroli disease
   b. Eagle-Barrett syndrome
   c. Byler disease
   d. Cystic fibrosis (CF)

8. A blind-ended structure which arises from the base of the cecum is known as the
   a. round ligament.
   b. appendix.
   c. duodenum.
   d. urethra.

9. To assess ureteropelvic junction obstruction, which ultrasound scan would you perform?
   a. Pelvis
   b. Renal
   c. Appendix
   d. Liver

10. Which is considered as the upper limit of the gallbladder wall with fasting?
    a. 0.5 mm
    b. 1 mm
    c. 2 mm
    d. 3 mm

Appendix

CHAPTER 1

1. c
2. b
3. c
4. c
5. Assessment notes, lab test results, correlating image modality study reports
6. Descriptions of ultrasound findings based on echo pattern and size, origin or location, number
7. Origin or location, number, size, and composition of abnormal findings
8. TO
9. CH
10. CH
11. TO
12. IR
13. IR
14. F
15. F
16. T
17. F
18. T
19. F

CHAPTER 2

1. c
2. d
3. b
4. a
5. c
6. a
7. c
8. d
9. c
10. b
11. c
12. a
13. d

CHAPTER 3

1. d
2. d
3. c
4. b
5. a
6. d
7. c
8. a
9. d
10. a
11. b
12. b
13. c

CHAPTER 4

1. b
2. d
3. a
4. d
5. b
6. Support cushion
7. Repetitive motions
8. Force
9. Abduction
10. cable support brace
11. ergonomics
12. For every 20 minutes of scan time look 20 feet away for 29 seconds.
13. 1. Pinch grip of the transducer. 2. Improper cable management. 3. Poor posture

CHAPTER 5

1. Hormones
2. endocrine system, target organs
3. pituitary gland, hypophysis
4. pituitary gland
5. pituitary gland, hypothalamus
6. Peristalsis
7. relaxed
8. contraction
9. lymphatic system
10. tendon
11. bones
12. ligaments
13. Hematopoiesis

CHAPTER 6

1. R
2. R
3. P
4. B
5. R
6. P
7. R
8. R
9. R
10. B
11. B
12. P
13. c
14. a
15. d
16. b
17. c
18. c
19. a
20. b

21. c
22. c

CHAPTER 7

1. c
2. d
3. b
4. a
5. d
6. a
7. d
8. b
9. c
10. c

CHAPTER 8

1. alanine aminotransferase (ALT); aspartate amino-transferase (AST)
2. International Organization for Standardization (ISO)
3. 10
4. 8
5. Prothrombin time (PT)
6. double
7. yolk sac; liver
8. lactic dehydrogenase (LD)
9. spinal tap
10. Cholesterol
11. muscle
12. blood

CHAPTER 9

1. b
2. c
3. F
4. F
5. T
6. T
7. T
8. F
9. F
10. T

CHAPTER 10

1. a
2. b
3. b
4. c
5. a
6. F
7. F
8. T
9. F
10. T

CHAPTER 11

1. F
2. T
3. F
4. F
5. IS
6. IS
7. LM
8. R
9. L
10. IS

CHAPTER 12

1. b
2. c
3. a
4. a
5. b
6. b
7. c
8. a
9. b
10. b

CHAPTER 13

1. b
2. d
3. c
4. F
5. T
6. F
7. T
8. T
9. F
10. T

CHAPTER 14

1. c
2. b
3. a
4. a
5. d
6. 2.0-3.0 cm
7. 1.5-2.5 cm
8. 2.0-3.0 cm
9. 1.0-2.0 cm
10. 12.0-18 cm

CHAPTER 15

1. D
2. B
3. A
4. C
5. E
6. F

7. F
8. T
9. F
10. F

CHAPTER 16

1. a
2. b
3. c
4. a
5. d
6. a
7. b
8. d
9. c
10. d

CHAPTER 17

1. c
2. d
3. E
4. F
5. C
6. A
7. H
8. G
9. D
10. B

CHAPTER 18

1. b
2. c
3. F
4. d
5. d
6. d
7. F
8. d
9. c
10. b

CHAPTER 19

1. b
2. c
3. a
4. c
5. d
6. T
7. F
8. T
9. F
10. F

CHAPTER 20

1. c
2. c
3. c
4. a
5. d
6. b
7. c
8. a
9. a
10. d
11. b
12. b
13. d
14. a

CHAPTER 21

1. d
2. b
3. d
4. b
5. a
6. a
7. b
8. c
9. c
10. c

CHAPTER 22

1. c
2. b
3. b
4. a
5. b
6. c
7. c
8. d
9. a
10. d

CHAPTER 23

1. b
2. a
3. c
4. b
5. 2
6. 2
7. 0
8. 2
9. 0
10. 2

CHAPTER 24

1. b
2. a
3. c
4. b
5. a
6. b
7. d
8. c
9. a
10. c

CHAPTER 25

1. c
2. c
3. b
4. a
5. c
6. b
7. b
8. b
9. b
10. a

CHAPTER 26

1. b
2. b
3. a
4. a
5. c
6. d
7. b
8. b
9. a
10. c

CHAPTER 27

1. E
2. G
3. H
4. F
5. A
6. J
7. C
8. D
9. B
10. I

CHAPTER 28

1. c
2. d
3. b
4. b

5. c
6. a
7. d
8. c
9. d
10. b

CHAPTER 29

1. b
2. a
3. a
4. d
5. c
6. b
7. b
8. d
9. a
10. c

CHAPTER 30

1. c
2. b
3. d
4. a
5. b
6. d
7. c
8. a
9. c
10. b

CHAPTER 31

1. b
2. c
3. d
4. a
5. d
6. a
7. c
8. b
9. d
10. b

CHAPTER 32

1. c
2. d
3. c
4. a
5. a
6. c
7. a
8. d
9. b
10. a

CHAPTER 33

1. b
2. c
3. a
4. b
5. d
6. T
7. F
8. F
9. F
10. T

CHAPTER 34

1. c
2. d
3. a
4. b

5. a
6. a
7. b
8. b
9. c
10. d

CHAPTER 35

1. c
2. b
3. b
4. a
5. b
6. b
7. d
8. b
9. b
10. d